SHANE O'MARA

Shane O'Mara is professor of Experimental Brain Research at Trinity College Dublin, the University of Dublin. He is principal investigator in, and was director of, the Trinity College Institute of Neuroscience, one of Europe's leading research centres for neuroscience, as well as being a Wellcome Trust senior investigator and a Science Foundation Ireland principal investigator. He is the author of *Why Torture Doesn't Work*, *A Brain for Business* and *In Praise of Walking*.

His musings on neuroscience, psychology and life can be found at the substack Brain Pizza.

ALSO BY SHANE O'MARA

SHANE O'MARA

Talking Heads

The New Science of How Conversation Shapes Our Worlds

VINTAGE

1 3 5 7 9 10 8 6 4 2

Vintage is part of the Penguin Random House group of companies
whose addresses can be found at global.penguinrandomhouse.com

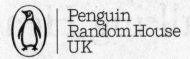

First published in Vintage in 2024
First published in Great Britain by The Bodley Head in 2023

penguin.co.uk/vintage

Printed and bound in Great Britain by Clays Ltd, Elcograf S.p.A.

The authorised representative in the EEA is Penguin Random House Ireland,
Morrison Chambers, 32 Nassau Street, Dublin D02 YH68

A CIP catalogue record for this book is available from the British Library

ISBN 9781529925579

Penguin Random House is committed to a sustainable future for
our business, our readers and our planet. This book is made from
Forest Stewardship Council® certified paper.

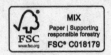

MIX
Paper | Supporting
responsible forestry
FSC
www.fsc.org
FSC® C018179

To Maura and Radhi, as usual, for everything . . . !

CONTENTS

AUTHOR'S NOTE

For my online writing, you can sign up via email at brainpizza.substack.com and get my writing that explores neuroscience, psychology and life delivered regularly to your inbox.

Mastodon: @shaneomara@mstdn.science
Instagram: @shanewriter

INTRODUCTION: WHAT HENRY TAUGHT US

In the early 1930s, a young boy had a bicycle accident. Except, perhaps he didn't. He might have fallen from his own bicycle; he might have been hit by someone else on a bicycle; he might have lost consciousness – or he might not have. The records are not clear. The records are also unclear on his age: he was, perhaps, six or seven years old. We do know that this accident happened – or didn't happen – in his hometown of Hartford, Connecticut, in the United States. The particulars can be only partially reconstructed; everyone's memories of the incident are vague, lost to time.[1]

The boy's medical records are equally vague, but X-rays from the time don't show any obvious brain injury. And yet, when he was ten, his epileptic fits started. Doctors wondered if these had anything to with the bicycle incident, but as it was unclear what – if anything – had happened, no one could say for sure. The occasional epileptic fits he suffered were mild at first, but increased in frequency and severity over the course of his teenage years. The drug treatments available didn't work, and his fits got worse as he grew older.

At this time, there was a little medical evidence to suggest that some forms of epilepsy could be controlled, or even abolished, by surgically removing a piece of brain tissue a bit larger than your middle finger: the hippocampal formation, about three or so centimetres from the skull, running approximately from the tip of your ear to your temple. Thinking at the time suggested that this part of the brain most likely had a role in smell, and perhaps also an unspecified role in emotion.[2] Perhaps, therefore, this was not really an important part of the brain, given the few things it seemed to be involved in.

The boy – by now a man aged twenty-seven – underwent an operation his surgeon described as 'frankly experimental' (for the surgeon had no idea if it would succeed in relieving the man's epileptic fits). The operation was performed on both sides of his brain (bilaterally), and the hippocampal formation was excised, along with some additional tissue (the amygdala). Some limited damage also occurred to one part of his frontal lobe.[3] The outcome of this 'frankly experimental' operation was remarkable. The man obtained almost immediate relief from his epileptic fitting, and his medication was substantially reduced. Moreover, his IQ remained normal and, in fact, seemed to rise slightly in the months after the operation – presumably because he was no longer taking powerful sedative drugs in an attempt to control his epilepsy. His general cognitive function did not change – that is to say, his ability to think, to turn something over in his mind, to recall old memories, to deliberately pay attention to something – all of these and related things seemed normal. His short-term memory also appeared normal: he could repeat back telephone numbers he had just heard, for example. But he couldn't learn a new telephone number off by heart to recall it on a later occasion.

It became obvious something was awry: the man seemed to have great trouble recalling new things that he had encountered in the course of daily life. His memory for the events of his daily life after the operation was lost – all because of the removal of two small pieces of brain tissue. This 'failed' operation pointed clearly to a brain region intimately involved in everyday learning and memory. This man was to become the most tested patient in history, meeting a large number of scientists whose identities remained opaque to him over the many years of psychological testing. He seemed to suffer from the most acute and profound case of amnesia – or loss of memory – ever recorded in the scientific literature. And this loss of memory did not recover through the next half-century of the man's life. The loss of memory was so devastating that he had to live in a protected community with carers, for he could no longer participate in everyday life – underlining the importance of memory for quotidian life. His identity was hidden in the scientific literature behind his initials: HM. Only after his death in 2007 was his real name – Henry Molaison – released.

Interestingly, Henry's profound amnesia did not preclude insight into his own condition, for many other aspects of his cognition, including his own thoughts regarding his own predicament, were relatively unaffected. He said of himself: 'Every day is alone in itself, whatever enjoyment I've had, and whatever sorrow I've had ... Right now, I'm wondering. Have I done or said anything amiss? You see, at this moment everything looks clear to me, but what happened just before? That's what worries me. It's like waking from a dream; I just don't remember.'[4] These sentences have always haunted me – they capture something of Henry's strobe-like, episodic existence. We all know what it is like to be present in a dream, to see, to feel, to know the dreamworld around you, only for it to dissipate, to slip out of reach, become lost to description, as we surface into consciousness. Imagine living a whole, long, adult life where everything that happens to you just slips away, leaving no trace behind. It's almost unthinkable, isn't it? Yet, for Henry, this became his whole life – his 'new normal'. And he was never to know of his scientific fame, or of the singular impact he had on how we think of the importance of particular brain regions for everyday memory. He changed a whole scientific field – the psychology and neuroscience of memory – and was completely oblivious to it. One point to emphasise here, which we will return to later, is that a life with such a profound amnesia means a life in the care of others. It could not be otherwise; carers provide the necessary memory scaffold for participating in everyday life. Full participation in the whole of our complex social lives depends on a normally functioning memory system.

This last consideration leads to a key idea: we so very often engage in remembering together. If one person is unable to remember anything, then cooperative efforts become fleeting or impossible. Imagine, for a moment, trying to create a sports team consisting of amnesiacs such as Henry. Team sports would be impossible, because Henry and his teammates would be unable to learn the rules of the game or to remember the set-piece drills they will have practised in order to counter the other team's plays. Henry was himself very cooperative, but building on these cooperative urges to engage in cooperative and complicated team sports would be difficult or impossible, especially if these efforts involve any complexity in terms of flexibility of rules to be applied during the game. This point generalises: without the easy, continuous and sophisticated application of memory to create shared realities together, creating complex social structures together becomes impossible.

Henry's case was not the first formal description of amnesia in the medical literature. There were some previous and somewhat overlooked cases, but these lacked a clear description of the underlying brain pathology. In 1878, many decades before Henry's case, the British neurologist Robert Lawson reported several cases of patients with amnesia resulting from alcohol abuse. Lawson's patients bear a striking similarity to Henry, because other aspects of their cognition seemed normal. Lawson, in summarising these cases, suggested that the 'feature of such cases which is sufficiently striking to give character to them is the almost absolute loss of memory for recent events. The patients are cheerful, attentive, understand what is said to them, and show little dementia as far as simple processes of reasoning are concerned.'[5]

Lawson wrote of one patient who was unable to remember

that her husband had died (her amnesia presumably arose from alcoholism). He noted that 'each time that the lamentable event was mentioned she regarded the information as something she had never heard before, and the grief she manifested was consistent with this remarkable forgetfulness. Still in other respects she was comparatively rational.'[6] Again, very much like Henry.

A few years after Lawson, the famous Russian neurologist Sergei Korsakoff wrote in a study of alcoholics with amnesia that 'especially characteristic is a derangement of memory and of the association of ideas'.[7] Today, people suffering from what is now called 'Korsakoff's syndrome' are known to have damage to a deep part of the brain (the anterior thalamus) which is closely interconnected with part of the hippocampal formation – damage to which was the source of Henry's amnesia.

It turns out, based on careful anatomical studies, that both the hippocampal formation and the anterior thalamus are in turn closely connected with the outermost layer of the brain – the cortex. To picture these brain regions, make a fist with your right hand, and place your left hand on top, covering the knuckles and right-hand thumb. Your covered thumb approximates the hippocampal formation, and the tip of your middle finger clenched against the palm of your hand approximates the anterior thalamus; the left hand approximates the cortex – the outer layer of the brain. Interactions between these areas give rise to memory.[8]

Korsakoff's syndrome patients suffer from a dense and unresolving amnesia, an amnesia similar to Henry's – but with a twist. Such patients may, unknowingly and unintentionally, tell untruths about themselves and others – they 'confabulate'.[9] (It is still unclear why Henry's case and similar cases of discrete hippocampal damage do not involve confabulation on top of their terrible amnesia.) One case study of confabulation in Korsakoff's syndrome concerns a patient with a severe mobility impairment caused by peripheral nerve damage who spent most of her time in a wheelchair. In response to the question 'What has happened to your feet?' she replied, incorrectly, 'A burning coal fell on my toes. I have lost two nails and now they are growing soft . . . now I need to put something very light on them.'[10] This answer makes a kind of sense – if a burning coal fell on your toes, then being confined to a wheelchair might be an outcome – but it was just not true. The patient had not been burned by coals at all, but had rationalised being in a wheelchair: for her, at least, this was a kind of an explanation, it felt like it might be true, it was possible, it might have happened.

Such patients seem to believe what they say, and may forget what they have said, once the conversation has passed. As one large-scale study of Korsakoff's patients concluded: the patients gave 'answers [that] were plausible and semantically appropriate, so that for an unfamiliar observer the confabulation was not obvious'.[11] Their answers are believable, and they seem to make sense – at least at that moment. This puts their unknowing conversational partner in a difficult position. Speak to them once, and all may seem fine; speak to them again and you could be told a completely different set of stories. You might, perhaps, conclude that they are liars (and not very good ones at that, because they have forgotten what they told you the last time) – or bullshitters, or worse, but they are not.[12]

Henry Molaison's case kicked off the modern era of the investigation of memory, and since then there has been remarkable progress by psychology and neuroscience in understanding how we tell each other the remembered stories of our lives. Henry's case became so central and important because it offered a clear and defined location in the brain supporting memory function. A torrent of research has followed. The circuits in the brain responsible for memory are now being illuminated in remarkable detail. Investigations into disorders of memory, such as might happen in cases of dementia, brain injury or stroke, are moving at such a rapid pace it is difficult to keep up. New and wonderful brain-imaging tools – allowing us to picture the working brain in flight – have been developed and are helping us to answer some of the oldest and most profound scientific questions regarding our astonishing memory capabilities.

In this book I will sometimes ask you as, a small experiment, to try to imagine what it is like to be without certain types of memory. This will be very hard for you to do. In essence, the challenge will be for you to imagine that you, too, have a profound amnesia – perhaps one extending backwards for a period of time (a 'retrograde' amnesia), or extending forward from a specific event and time, such as a brain injury (an 'anterograde' amnesia). For example, think about the most important people in your personal life: perhaps your spouse, perhaps your children, perhaps your parents, perhaps a person for whom you have unrequited love (or, indeed, hatred – the nature of the feeling doesn't really matter), or perhaps a work colleague. Now, imagine that all the knowledge you have of all these people goes *poof* – somehow it disappears. This, of course, is not fanciful, for it happens to countless people in a gradual fashion every day, through ageing, neurodegenerative diseases and other processes.

To help you imagine what life with amnesia is like, just think about all the people we meet, talk with and forget over the course of the years: we forget them through a subtle, amnesia-like process. Find a picture of the kids you were at school with – these crop up on social media, or perhaps you might have an old school yearbook. Perhaps you were in a class of twenty or so children. You sat beside them every day for years, you fought with them, you played with them, you were friends with them, they called around to your house to play games, you were on teams with them. But putting the names to the faces several years or decades on is difficult for many people – you find you have forgotten your classmates' names, and new people have come along who have taken their place. I continue to be personally mortified when I think back to when I met a classmate a few years ago in a mutual friend's house who greeted me, without hesitation, by name – a classmate whom I sat beside for certain classes in school – and of whom I had no explicit recall at all.

You might find remembering those long-forgotten classmate names a little easier if you take the photograph and if you work at *remembering together* with someone from that class whom you are still friends with. This is known as 'collaborative' remembering,[13] where people work together to piece together knowledge in common, knowledge previously on the tip of their tongue – because, of course, at the age of seven or eight you knew the names of everybody in your class, and now you've forgotten the names of most of them. (Happily, our mutual friend saw my discomfort and dropped my former classmate's name into the conversation – it helped, a bit.) Collaborative memory is complex: each partner will likely recall at least a little of what the other partner recalls, but when the partners are probed and tested together, richer and deeper memories result. Conversational exchanges and discussions can result in a shared, cooperative memory search superior to recall that is conducted alone (as my friend's intervention to cue my memory shows).

Another way memory loss happens is when people are struck by one of the several, terrible varieties of dementia, where they can lose all sorts of memories: autobiographical information about themselves, biographical details about others, information about the world at large. Life for the person with dementia gradually empties of colour and detail. Gaps appear in their conversation, as they lose the thread of the tête-à-tête. Gradually, insidiously, their condition worsens, and they may begin to fail to recognise the people they know and love; their minds gradually seem to become blanker, with no thoughts coming to mind, or if thoughts are articulated, they are usually thoughts about the immediate *here and now* – the person becomes ever more trapped in a continual present, unable to make the mental journeys along the timelines to an imagined future or an experienced past.

Now, imagine a society where everyone at large is afflicted with a condition like this: a world populated by Henry Molaisons. How can the members of that society learn about and understand the world around them? The answer is obvious: they cannot. Their society – with its signs, symbols, rituals, norms, shared under-standings, rules, procedures, records – will be forever lost. We depend on memory, all of the time, to make our complex, social lives possible.

*

We have seen that amnesia devastates a person's ability to learn new things, and may even affect their recall of old things. It would seem, therefore, that the purpose of the amazing memory systems of our brain is to allow us to recall the past. Cases such as Henry's, or those described by Lawson, seem to demand this interpret-ation. Remember, though, the past may not all be gone. There might be little to no retrograde – or backward-facing – amnesia. Rather, there might be anterograde – or forward-facing – amnesia where the largely automatic learning and then remembering of newly encountered events and things is lost. But another view of memory is possible too, a more expansive one than recording and recalling our everyday experiences. A more expansive view might suggest, for example, that our memories evolved to allow us to use our past experiences (including very recent past experiences) to respond to the demands of the present time and place. A simple example: you meet some new colleagues at work, learn about them and what they'll be doing, and remember who they are the next time you meet them. We can go further, though: for memories also allow us to imagine alternative times and places, to conjure up possible future events in our heads and then share these imagined future events with others in conversation.

Henry, for example, could not use information from his recent past to interpret his present. He met the late neuroscientist Suzanne Corkin on hundreds of occasions from the early 1960s through to his death in 2007. He never remembered her name and could not tell who she was.[14] Each time they met, a social connection had to be established afresh: a social connection lasting for the testing session, and a social connection which was lost – for Henry – once they were finished. Similarly, Henry showed an impoverished imagination regarding the future – he was not really able to conjure up the richly imagined alternative futures that we do all the time.

Antoine Roquentin, the central character in Jean-Paul Sartre's famous 1938 existentialist novel *Nausea* (*La Nausée*), declares that 'a man is always a teller of tales, he lives surrounded by his stories and the stories of others, he sees everything that happens to him through them; and he tries to live his own life as if he were telling a story'. Sartre's intuition, voiced through Roquentin, is correct. When you meet a friend, you share stories about what you've been doing or what you intend to do. As we shall see, you shape the story according to the listeners present, and this in turn can affect what you remember. Our memories are consistently used socially to fill out, shape and enrich the gossip, stories and conversations we have with others. When Henry met Suzanne Corkin, he didn't have the regularly updated stock of gossip, stories and conversations that he might have had, had he not suffered from a terrible and deep amnesia.

However, this continual interchange of stories and conversations with others brings a certain hazard: our memories are subtly tweaked and updated by our conversations with other people. As we shall see, our memories are a multi-layered record, subtly overwritten and updated on the fly as we converse within our social groups – and all without our realising that this delicate overwriting has occurred. And because of the fragility of human memory, others might misremember or misattribute what we have said – as the legendary American baseball player, manager and coach Yogi Berra famously put it, 'I never said most of the things I said,' meaning others misremembered what Berra (supposedly) had said, and misattributed these misrememberings to him. This malleability of memory means we must, and do, learn from our earliest years to trust what we are told by others[15] – we simply do not expect to be routinely and treacherously lied to during our everyday lives. In fact, what we hear in the course of our everyday lives when talking to each other tends to be true, or we usually accept it as true[16] (this why there will always be con artists and grifters able to part people from their money – trusting marks are easy money for the con artist).

We use memory effortlessly in conversation – telling our truths to others – for revealing information about yourself smooths your conversational path with the other speaker. Conversation emerges from a continuous dialogue between your brain systems supporting memory and language, duelling, or aligning, with the brain systems supporting memory and language of another person. Duelling because we might be arguing about something; aligning because we are agreeing about something. We expect conversation to involve talking about ourselves to others, when we will make many personal disclosures, and, reciprocally, we expect others to talk about themselves to us. And so central is information exchange to daily life that we use your refusal to offer information about yourself as negative evidence regarding the kind of person you might be. Being unwilling to talk about yourself is an unwelcome experience for others. During conversation we don't like other people to be tight-lipped, closed off, excessively circumspect: social life hinges on conversation – but conversation obeying the convention that we try to avoid lying or speaking without any regard to the truth (bullshitting, which too often degrades and pollutes our world).[17] Truth matters in our everyday lives.

We tell what we know to others, and (generally speaking) we believe what others say. What they say then becomes part of us, for it is woven into the connections – the synapses – between our brain cells. And all of these conversations become part of what we think, remember and imagine; they become part of our own personal narrative; and they become part of what we tell others in conversation.

Most of us, from childhood onwards, invest our trust in what others say. We're not unbiased in this; we have favourites. We listen to – and learn from – friends, family, teachers, celebrities. And we do this for good reason: this is how we survive and prosper in our complex social groups. You ignore at your peril the elder who says 'Do not eat those bright yellow berries.' And, in turn, we learn, remember and readily transmit this information to others. Trusting in what others say, and subsequently incorporating what others say into our memories, allows us to live our interdependent, hyper-social lives and sustain our restless and complex social worlds. These ideas help unpack further the psychological mechanisms supporting the larger-scale creation of shared institutions and organisations and the collective cognitive artefact of the nation.

It is often said that seeing is believing, but 'sharing is believing' too.[18] The concept of 'sharing is believing' emphasises that people adjust their communication to align with their partner's attitudes, which also affects what they remember. The Columbia University psychologist Tory Higgins and his colleagues have considered the issue of how we come to create shared realities – how we come to believe the same things, and act together on those beliefs:[19] recall our imagined elder's admonition, 'Do *not* eat those yellow berries!' Higgins and his colleagues define a shared reality as a 'perceived commonality of inner states (feeling, beliefs, and concerns about the world) with other people'.[20] They add that the major building block of shared reality is 'sharing is believing': I share my knowledge about the poisonous yellow berries with you, and you tell others in turn about how dangerous they are. This idea reflects themes expressed throughout this book. In conversation, we generally reveal ourselves – what we're thinking, what we're feeling – to other individuals quickly and without much of an effort to truly hide what we really think or feel (unless hiding it matters in some way, in which case we dissimulate, shape our responses to who we're talking to or straightforwardly lie to them).

We humans are naturally motivated to create a shared reality with others, based on shared feeling, beliefs and concerns about the world. This shared reality helps us to build social connections and understanding with each other (unless you are paranoid, in which case building these connections will be difficult, or even denied you, because of your distrust and disbelief in what others say). Indeed, people who are routinely sceptical of the assertions of their friends and other conversational partners tend to be somewhat ostracised within the conversational group. We look askance at the untrusting paranoid, forever glancing over their shoulder, certain that they alone see some far-reaching truth denied the rest of us, questioning with unnecessary hostility everything said to them.[21] Conversations with the corrosively conspiracy-minded are impossible to navigate, with their doom loops of circular logic, unmoored from the empirical world – whether their focus is as relatively harmless as UFOs or as deadly as the anti-vaxxers.[22] Happily, there are few of them, and even if social media has amplified the sound of their voices, they seem not to be increasing in number.[23]

We use group conversation to constantly recalibrate what it is that we know about our world, and to set the boundaries of what is reasonable to discuss within that world. Within our groups we have what we might refer to loosely as 'collective memories' – memories for things that we, the members of our in-groups, know in common, and that are not shared by those not of our groups, or of our tribes, or indeed of our nations. Moreover, our shared collective memories only really apply to our specific community or group, and that is where they exert their most meaningful purchase on the popular imagination.[24]

My retelling my community's collective memories to a non-community member might be interesting to that non-member – in a kind of an anthropological sense – but is not likely to really galvanise them into action. Imagine two travellers striking up a conversation in an airport; both are heading home for Christmas. One traveller is from a small town with a tradition of decorating the main street with a particular style and type of Christmas lights, and then celebrating the turning on of the lights with particular events, and this tradition has been passed down for generations. The other traveller – a non-community member – may find this tradition a little bit interesting and (just about) worth learning about, but it is not likely to galvanise them to change their travel plans and visit the small town, despite the other traveller's enthusiasm and entreaties, because they do not have a personal connection to the community or to the events being discussed. One person is passing time in conversation; the other is reliving past events in conversation. For whom are the small-town Christmas lights more alive?

Imagining alternatives, learning from what others say and telling others what we know allow us to construct shared, communal and collective *cognitive* realities. These shared realities can be small-scale – from romantic relationships to family ties – or they can be much larger and more abstract. In this book I will discuss how our memories are transmitted from one person to another through conversation, and how this person-to-person transmission allows us to learn from each other quickly and easily. This person-to-person transmission forms the basis of the social and cultural practices binding us to our larger social groups and committing us to the large-scale, imagined communities comprising our nations. Memories and conversation allow us to build friendships and groups, teams and organisations, institutions and nations; and the existence of all these communities, large and small, is dependent on the joint and collective exercise of memory and imagination, where we muse about the past, present and future and engage in the shared enterprise of selecting our future journeys together.[25]

A central implication is that our nations are *imagined*: they are shared realities created by human thought, imagination and action: there is no inscribed tablet given to us from on high, naming and numbering all of the nations of the world, unchanging, for all time. Nations have been transformed through time, because of geography, military might and colonialism, among other factors.

Even now, there are factions and groups wanting to create new nations, perhaps a group within a specific geographical region who aspire to establishing a separate nation, independent from the one to which they currently belong, a nation they *imagine* and want to bring to life. Our imaginations can lead us to engage in violence and murder: wars of conquest and domination (as Russia is currently undertaking in Ukraine). But our imaginations, generously exercised, can have peaceful and prosperous outcomes too, where nations come together to work together for their own good and for the good of others.

Beyond nations, we humans have imagined into being even more abstract supranational entities of varying power, scale and reach, such as the United Nations, the Olympic Games, the World Health Organisation and so many more. Because nations (and indeed international organisations) are *imagined entities*, because they do not exist as Platonic ideals, objectively, outside and beyond human cognition, memory and imagination, we are left with an interesting paradox: the nations of the world are cognitively arbitrary, but they are also reasonably cognitively stable entities with which to organise our human affairs.

And without memory – as happens in conditions causing amnesia – these multiple, shared, social, cultural possibilities are utterly obviated. They are simply not possible. Memories achieve these astonishing things – from binding us together in groups to building our nations together – because they reach deep into the recesses of our brains, changing many of us, or all of us, along with our perceptions of the world around us, at the same time.

Of all the millions of species on our planet, we humans are unique in forming these shared realities on which we depend to live our lives. Moreover, these shared realities depend on the normal functioning of brain systems supporting cognition and memory but exercised together. The shared realities are built upon the common biology of many different brains drawing on similar cognitive capacities to remember and imagine things afresh *together* – and very frequently so in storytelling and conversation. Our brains allow unique repurposing and promiscuous interactions between differing brain systems. This is our killer app: the way our brain mixes together differing cognitive functions, allowing new abilities to emerge that would otherwise be dormant.

Our conversations and stories allow us to extend our very *selves* – our thoughts, our hopes, our memories, our dreams, our desires – into the fabric and function of each other's brains. And the same is true of others: the thoughts, memories and conversations of other people are in our heads in the most intimate and private way imaginable, for these thoughts, memories and conversations change the very fabric of our brains, rewriting and redirecting the course of our own thoughts, memories and imagination. This way of thinking about memory – one going far beyond regarding it as a psychological faculty simply serving recall of the past – turns how we think about human memory inside out, taking our memories from inside our brains and dropping them directly in the world beyond our bodies, where memories play their central role during the conversations, gossip and stories we continually exchange with each other.

This is why memories acquire such power: the power to redirect what we think and feel, and thereby to make and break our social groups, organisations, institutions, nations.

*

In this book I will sometimes draw upon on two commonly used distinctions regarding memory. Psychology has borrowed the term 'autobiography' from literature and appended it to memory, giving us the portmanteau 'autobiographical memory'. As you might imagine, these memories are records of the events of your life. 'Semantic memory', on the other hand, is your knowledge of the general facts of the world, devoid of any autobiographical component: things like the names of the continents or the colours of national flags.

Another phrase we will encounter repeatedly here is 'default mode'. This is used widely in information technology and computer programming: the default mode is something a system or process is designed to go to automatically. A common example is a video game automatically starting on the first level of the game – the default level – unless a different level is selected or a bypass is possible. Our brain also has a default mode: it approximates to the experience of 'mind wandering', which, despite its name, is not idle time at all. Mind wandering involves coursing backwards and forwards through the big picture of our lives and then zooming in on details. While doing so, we reflect on our past, present and future: we cycle through thoughts concerning our lives – powered along by our memories. Mind wandering allows us to see both the forest and the trees of our intense social lives. When we have downtime, and our smartphones are inaccessible, we default into more or less this style of thinking without really intending to. Current estimates suggest that we might spend as much as 40% of our time in this mind-wandering state, paradoxically combining behavioural quiescence with furious mental activity. Because the process of mind wandering, big-picture thinking and musing on our social lives is such a pervasive mental activity and involves so much of the brain system, it is thought to be the default mode of brain function.[26] Our brains are very busy when we are apparently doing nothing; but we are not doing nothing – we are trying to sort out what's going on with our lives!

Autobiographical memory and semantic memory work seamlessly together – usually. Sometimes these types of memory break down, and break down quite badly. Imagine, for a moment, that you suffer from autobiographical and semantic amnesia. You would be without memory of your personal past, and you would find that your knowledge of the world around you is also lost. You can still speak, and you can still think. If asked what is on your mind at present, sitting there in your chair, what would you say? There are very few possibilities. One is that you would be thinking about nothing at all – you would be mentally blank – for nothing comes to mind, as there are no thoughts and memories sliding in and out of your consciousness for you to consider, to use, to dismiss. Another possibility is that you would simply report your present sensations, just the things you are currently thinking and feeling, seeing and hearing; your inner world would approximate your outer world as interpreted by your various senses. Your experience of daily life would be a succession of unconnected episodes – it would be as if you were somehow living your life in strobe, with little connection or continuity between one moment and the next.

Our inner mental world is normally a world of abstraction – one where we humans engage in mental time travel, coursing forward in our heads to imagined futures, backward to past events, and re-centring ourselves again in the present moment, to talk with others and reimagine together our future plans. Living with amnesia – living, effectively, in strobe – means you have no personal mental extension through time, for you are unable to seamlessly revisit your past life and experiences, and you are unable to journey forward in time to your imagined future lives or worlds. This is one price we pay if we have amnesia.

The shared worlds we hope to create in the future are, necessarily, worlds of the imagination – we travel to them in our minds, create stories and songs about them, and perhaps even devise the technology to make them happen. And we can cherish great and fantastical ambitions. Albert Einstein, at the age of sixteen, imagined running through space to catch up with a beam of light, intuiting that it would be an electromagnetic wave at rest.[27] This imaginative skill is a most remarkable capacity, one dependent in the most intimate and personal way on the integrity and reliability of the brain systems responsible for memory and imagination. Alexander the Great, king of Macedonia in the fourth century BC, on seeing the breadth and extent of his domain allegedly 'wept, seeing as he had no more worlds to conquer'.[28] What a foreclosing of his imagination if this were true. But we do continuously imagine new worlds to conquer. More recently, David Bowie wondered in song if there was life on Mars; and a few decades later the billion-aire Elon Musk hopes to colonise this near-earth, red-hued world.

*

This book starts with how and why we humans talk to each other and ends with the vast, shared, imagined realities that are our nations. A neuroscience of nation building may seem a stretch, but, as I will show, nations are ultimately built by brains. Yet, as we shall see, our thoughts, memories and imaginings are much more than in our heads; in fact, I will claim that all our nations – every single one of them – began as conversations about what might come to be – the exercise of our imaginations, extended forward in time.

I hope you will forgive me for simplifying certain things and simply skating past others; any errors and omissions, while unin-tentional, are certainly my own. To reuse a famous and well-worn phrase, I have tried to keep things as simple as possible, but not simpler. The neuroscientific and psychological literatures treat-ing, for example, mental time travel, learning, memory and cognition are almost incomprehensibly large. Similarly, there are extensive literatures in sociology, history, geography, anthropol-ogy and political science speaking to some of the arguments of this book. Writing a thematically wide-ranging book becomes an exer-cise in exclusion. The writing must stop somewhere.

1.
HAVING CONVERSATIONS
WITH OTHERS

One of life's great pleasures is running into an old friend or acquaintance and chatting idly about the past, present and future. It can be disconcerting to realise that that unpleasant kid from your schooldays is no longer present: they have grown up and so have you, and you discover this how? By talking to each other, and in that momentary conversation a relationship might be transformed for the better and memories of the past updated, or even overwritten entirely. A conversation is exactly that: a dialogue – not a monologue – and it requires turn taking. One person speaks, then stops at the right moment, and the other person speaks, then stops, allowing the other person back in to speak – a game of verbal ping-pong with turn taking as its foundation.

Conversation is a form of multi-tasking, because you are running several psychological processes at once: comprehension of words and sentences, at the same time as producing speech. When saying a word like 'cat', the muscles in the mouth and throat must be precisely coordinated to produce the sounds of the individual letters in the correct order. The brain must plan the muscle movements, very rapidly and ahead of time, and execute the muscle movements in a coordinated manner. This means speaking is highly complex, and involves the coordinated movement of multiple muscles in the face, jaw, tongue and larynx. This process is called motor programming, and it includes the planning, execution and coordination of muscle movements.

Finally, we must understand what is said to us; but language comprehension is not a purely auditory affair. We use other types of information to understand the spoken language of other people. Ambiguous speech sounds are sounds that are produced similarly but have different meanings – such as the sounds 'p' and 'b', or the words 'pat' and 'bat'. Such sounds can be hard to understand if you are listening in difficult conditions (on the phone or in a noisy environment). In this case, we also rely upon cues from the lips and mouth (such as their shape, emphasis and enunciation), and indeed the body language and gestures of the other person, to comprehend fully what it is that they are saying.

Language is certainly one of the defining characteristics of what it is to be human, even though languages differ in all sorts of ways across cultures and even within cultures. As the noted British psycholinguist Stephen Levinson and his colleague Francisco Torreira point out, the rapid exchange of short spells of conversation is one aspect of language use similar across all languages.[1] Typically, conversational interchanges are of a few seconds' duration for both speakers, though obviously there is considerable variation in this, not least because some people just drone on seemingly without end.

Here's an imagined conversation about *Mary Poppins*, the movie, with my smartphone-stopwatch-estimated speaking times:

Person 1: 'Hey, have you seen *Mary Poppins* recently?' (3 secs)
Person 2: 'Yeah, streamed it last night. One of my faves.' (3 secs)
Person 1: 'Me too! I love Mary Poppins, she's so magical and kind.' (3 secs)

Person 2: 'Oh yeah? My favourite is Bert, with his terrible
cockney accent!' (5 secs)

Person 1: 'Yeah, I like him too. But I love the Banks children
as well.' (5 secs)

Person 2: 'Yeah, they're great. But I gotta go now, sorry.'
(3 secs)

Person 1: 'Have you ever noticed how the different songs
in the movie reflect the characters' emotions? Pretty
clever, I think.' (6 secs)

Person 2: 'Yeah, no, but sorry gotta go – my bus is coming.
Catch you again.' (3 secs)

This little interchange illustrates these points: there's an
opener question, a little bit of back-and-forth evoking different
characters, a sticking to the joint conversation topic (thereby sharing a particular reality for a moment), a small bit of droning, an
attempt to exit the conversation by Person 2, a little more droning,
and then, finally, a successful extrication from the conversation by
Person 2. And baked into the conversation is the shared reality of
having seen the same movie, recall of the individual characters
and preferences noted for the different characters, and the attempt
to get away from the conversation. Conversations are complicated happenings when you look at them a little more closely.
Turn taking in conversation implies considerable neural machinery supporting simultaneous language production and language
comprehension in both listener and speaker.

We generally have no memory of how we learned to speak in
our early years, nor do we have any recall of those early infant
moments where, seemingly helpless, we tried to communicate our
needs and wants without having words to deploy. Even then,
though, we weren't entirely helpless – we cried, we giggled, we
gooed, we rolled our eyes, we puckered our nose and lips, leading
our caregivers to respond quickly to our needs. And this period of
apparent helplessness is an essential part of development, crucial

for mastering the art of conversation at the heart of our social lives. Long periods of mutual back-and-forth between carer and child form the building blocks of turn taking. Turn taking emerges early in the first few weeks of life, where infants respond to and initiate eye contact and gesture at the appropriate points of communication with a caregiver.[2] Thus we can surmise that turn taking is innate – it is inborn. Moreover, sign language follows the same rules that apply to spoken languages. Signers initiate and terminate during the taking of turns in signed conversations with the same temporal gaps that are observed in spoken language.[3] During an average day we spend perhaps several hours in turn taking, engaging in as many as 1,500 such turn takings during our waking hours.[4]

Many of these turn takings occur as we face each other, an orientation where gesture and gaze make sense, because we can look into the eyes and observe the hand movements of the other person. We can more deeply mind-read the other person, because we have much more information to work from – we can quickly and easily infer from the emphatic gestures they make, the tempo of their movements, the flickering movements of their eyes, the bobbing and nodding of their head, just how emotionally engaged and invested they are in what they're talking about. Turn taking does not depend solely on the language system of the brain *per se*, but is built deeply into our systems of communication, be they gestural or spoken.

Let's think about a short, conversational interchange – this could be by telephone, by video call or in person. The conversation consists of short bursts of questions, statements, autobiographical reveals, replies, generally related to the topic under discussion. Imagine you're speaking with your doctor, who says, 'Hi, how are you? It's been a month since I saw you last,' and you reply quickly, 'I'm actually feeling quite well. I think the medication is doing the trick.' The doctor asks, 'No side effects? No unpleasant pains?' and you say, 'No, actually, none whatsoever.' The doctor replies,

'That's good. We can start to taper you off the medication in a little while.'

Let's draw out the role of memory in this conversation: you must *remember* to go to your doctor at the right time for your appointment; you must *remember* how medication is affecting you; and you must respond to the doctor's questions regarding side effects (do you remember what these are? Or are you guessing?). The doctor must *recall* who you are and what was the matter with you, *remember* what the prescription was (or *remember* to look the prescription up in the patient records), and then *remember* to gently drive the conversation to discover if the treatment is working (and *remember* to ask about any side effects). And the doctor must repeat this process with other patients, perhaps four or five times per hour, over the course of a day and not make mistakes, while remaining pleasant and in the moment for each patient. This requires the repeated interrogation of memory systems in two separate heads, focused and synchronised around the medical problem, just as both patient and doctor deploy their memory systems for face recognition, voice recognition and the recognition of emotions; and the doctor must have empathy for the pain or suffering the patient might be feeling. Moreover, both patient and doctor must find common expression and understanding in the conversation. Afterwards, some of the details of the encounter will remain sticky in the heads of the doctor and patient, details to be recalled from memory and then discussed on the next visit.

Underlying this conversation is the speed and rapidity of the turn taking from speaker to speaker – doctor to patient, patient to doctor. The gap between one speaker ceasing to speak and the next speaker starting to speak is typically about a fifth of a second (200 milliseconds).[5] We are responding during conversation about as quickly as it is possible for us to respond:[6] indeed we are responding so fast that it is 'close to the minimal reaction time to a starting gun'.[7] Yet we are responding to a conversation – something more complicated than the straightforward stimulus of the report of a starting pistol.

The units of conversational turns tend to be of a fixed size during ordinary conversation – we tend to speak for approximately two seconds or so at a time, but, clearly, there is lots of variation. Turn taking minimises the overlap between the speech streams of the two individuals participating in the conversation.[8] Nor do you need, necessarily, to see the person to whom you are speaking to interject into the conversation at the appropriate time – we do it all the time during ordinary telephone calls. And, of course, people with visual impairments can participate fully in conversations, too. Minimising the overlap is a standard rule in conversation. One person talking over another is experienced by other listeners as unpleasant and highly discordant. Talking over someone doesn't win you the battle of words, although it might allow you to talk out the clock without having given an answer. The impression you have given to listeners may not be what you want it to be – you'll be seen, perhaps, as self-important, and as a bit of a jerk:

> Business consultant: 'So, have you ever thought about how the economy is just like a game of chess? I mean, you have to be strategic, and you have to think ahead, and plan all your moves.'
>
> Client: 'I was hoping to tell you about the problems I'm having with managing our cash flow.'
>
> Business consultant: 'Yeah, yeah, that's great, but let me just finish this thought. So, the economy is like chess, and you have to be smart about it.'
>
> Client: 'Can I just talk about our cash flow?'
>
> Business consultant: 'Oh, sure, sure, go ahead. But let me just riff on this chess-economy thing first. It'll help you think a bit more clearly about your cash-flow issues.'
>
> Client: 'Can you please stop interrupting me? I'm trying to talk about my business and you're not even listening.'

Business consultant: 'Oh, yeah, cash flow. Yeah, chess. I'm
   just trying to explain how the economy works, it's not
   that complicated, once you get what chess is about.'
Client: 'I think we're done here. You're not listening – cash
   flow is my problem. I've been here twenty minutes, and
   all you're talking about is chess.'
Business consultant: 'I'm just trying to help, you know.
   Chess, you know. The economy, you know. It's not hard
   to understand.'

Some teeth grinding, and the client leaves.

I think it's pretty clear who the unpleasant person is in this
exchange. Moreover, they are uninformed too – the economy is
not like a game of chess – and just because they love their stupid
idea doesn't mean anyone else will. Reading the reactions of others
to what you say is also a vital conversational skill.

Languages may have many tens of thousands or more words,
with an associated grammar; the words must be articulated in a
fashion allowing you to get going quickly when it is your turn. You
must comprehend and predict what it is the person is saying to
you while they are speaking, and do so at great speed. Around the
one-second mark into a two-second speech utterance, we have
predicted what the response, the content and the intentions of the
other person will be, even if we don't yet know if the statement is
going to end in a question, an offer, a request or whatever.

The evidence suggests that the last common ancestor of we
humans and our Neanderthal relatives had a vocal tract and associated physiology and genetics to support the use of speech,[9]
implying that the origins of turn taking are evolutionarily ancient.
Neanderthals could probably engage in signed or gestural communication using their hands, and were almost certainly capable of
engaging in spoken language.[10] These capacities imply a very considerable cognitive capacity not apparent in our close primate
relatives (who nonetheless develop turn taking during vocal

exchanges early in life).[11] The neural and psychological roots of our language, memory and movement systems work together, allowing quick and easy communication of our mental states – and these roots are very ancient indeed.

*

The neuroscientist Sara Bögels of Radboud University in Nijmegen in the Netherlands has been investigating what goes on in the brain during turn taking in ordinary conversation, while also trying to simultaneously measure what is happening in the brain.[12] To simulate regular conversation, Bögels used long and short forms of the same kinds of questions – such as the alternative forms 'So you play volleyball?' or 'So you play volleyball on Thursday night?' She also measured the electrical activity of the brain of the listener (the electroencephalogram or EEG) during the asking of these questions to get a sense of the critical points in the questions the brain responded to. To test the brain responses, she had people rate the questions and come to a consensus about the word at which the answer could be predicted.[13] Bögels found, as Levinson had also suggested, that conversational turn taking happened quickly, usually with a 200-millisecond break, and, crucially, that signals could be found in the brain showing that answer preparation happened early in the question, after the first couple of words, rather than later, when the question had been asked.

Thus, we prepare answers easily and quickly based on our anticipation of what the end of the question will be (of course, we don't always get this right, especially if there's a mismatch between what we know, what we think the other person knows and what they end up saying). We understand conversation quickly because we anticipate or predict the likely future content of a sentence during a conversation. This means we track the dynamics of the spoken words in those sentences (by 'dynamics' I mean the length of words, the intensity with which they are spoken, their difference and similarity to other words, and understanding them against a perhaps ambiguous, noisy background). The way our brain processes spoken language can be contrasted with how it processes individual sounds. By comparing how we understand the meaning of a spoken word, such as the word 'cat', with how we understand the sound of a cat meowing, we can demonstrate that the brain processes spoken language more efficiently. Similarly, if we compare our understanding of the word 'laughter' to the sound of laughter, we can see that the brain is able to understand the meaning of the spoken word much faster than it can understand the sound itself. This highlights the ability of the brain to quickly decode and understand the meaning of spoken language. The brain decodes (or understands) the spoken word ('cat') more quickly than it decodes the sound equivalent (meowing) – measured using a special brain-imaging technique known as magnetoencephalography, or MEG, because it measures to the millisecond the brain at work.[14] The brain tracks the sounds of words accurately in time and decodes them more quickly than sounds corresponding to the word, because spoken words have primacy for humans, and human speech is special for the human brain, compared to other sounds.

Findings like these are suggestive, but we can go further to show that speech is special for the brain hearing it. One way to do this is to set the listener up to expect a particular word to complete a sentence, and then present them with that word, or a different word, or degraded or somewhat masked versions of those words.[15] The idea is that recognising words may involve the rapid comparison of predicted (the words you expect you're going to hear) and heard speech (the words you actually hear) sounds, and that noting the difference in the comparison (formally, 'prediction error') is how we figure out what is being said. Some words can sound ambiguous because they share similar first syllables. 'Hygiene' and 'hijack', for example, should increase prediction error and hence brain activity only at later time points when different segments are predicted ('-giene' versus '-jack'). There was delayed recognition of the actually heard words (such as 'hygiene') after hearing a neighbouring, closely related word ('hijack') several minutes earlier; the brain shows greater activity when words were recognised after we heard their distinctive sounds, but not before. However, this effect was not present for non-words ('higent'). In other words, we continuously update our understanding of the words we hear based on how well they match what we expected to hear.

Conversations often open with, or contain, questions. It's sometimes thought that the way we phrase the questions we put to others can have an impact on the answers they give to us. An example to illustrate this idea: if I ask for your opinion on whether brie is a cheese or not, I can ask the question indirectly by saying 'Some people think brie is not a cheese – what do you think?' or directly by saying 'Do you think brie is a cheese or not?' This subtle difference in the way the question is worded may influence your response. The question couched in indirect language allows you more freedom to give your honest opinion, rather than being prompted to agree or disagree with a stated belief. Where you ask the question directly, you don't hint at the views that might be held elsewhere by other people. Thus the difference in phrasing might affect the opinion that you offer in response.

How people respond to these different types of questions has been studied by the psychologists David Scott Yeager and Jon Krosnick of Stanford University,[16] especially differing types of indirect versus direct questions. For example, if adolescents are asked the question 'Some people have lots of friends and others have few friends – which are you?', as opposed to 'Do you have lots of friends?', they find no difference between the direct and indirect phrasing of the questions, despite the indirect question purportedly placing a greater cognitive load on you when you must think about the answer. A reasonable conclusion from Yeager and Krosnick is that direct versus indirect questions really don't make much difference. That would be the wrong conclusion, because the way you ask questions can have an impact on the answers you receive, and this impact is determined by the group of people you are asking and their level of understanding and knowledge on the subject. The way you phrase your questions for a survey on recycling should align with the knowledge and understanding of the population you are questioning. You would not ask complex technical questions of school children, or pose very basic recycling questions to your local green party members. Moreover, the questions you ask should align with the knowledge you assume your participants have on the subject, and their ability to answer the questions in a way that provides the information you are looking for. The participants might not have the knowledge you expect, even though you might – incorrectly – believe they do.

How you are asked questions, and in what order, really matters, because the way you probe your own memory in response to questions changes depending on the way you are asked particular questions. The psychologist Francis Huang of the University of Missouri has been concerned with studying the effects of bullying on children and adults over many years. In an especially important paper, he and his colleague Dewey Cornell find that the order of questions has a marked effect on whether or not children report themselves as victims of bullying.[17] More precisely, they find that when surveying children, asking specific questions about particular incidents of bullying leads children to report that they have been bullied, whereas asking general questions does not. Remarkably, providing a definition of bullying (defined as the 'repeated use of one's strength or popularity to injure, threaten, or embarrass another person on purpose. [It] can be physical, verbal, or social'), and asking children if they have been bullied using that definition leads to a massive under-reporting of bullying – children typically report not having been bullied. Students were asked specific questions related to four examples of different types of bullying (physical, verbal, social and cyber bullying): they were asked if they had experienced these forms of bullying in the current school year. Providing specific examples of bullying (such as

'Verbal bullying involves repeatedly teasing, putting down, or insulting someone on purpose. I have been verbally bullied at school this year'), rather than wide-ranging bullying-victimisation statements (such as 'I have been bullied at school'), results in an enormous increase (ranging from 29% to 76%, depending on the survey) in victimisation rates. The type of memory probe matters: surveys asking general-to-specific questions seem to substantially under-report bullying, whereas asking specific questions and moving to more general questions seems to be a better strategy for probing recall. Thus the way questions are asked greatly influences the accuracy of the information obtained: asking specific questions and then moving to general questions is usually better. Our recall is shaped by the way we are questioned.

*

Although culture is sticky, it can and does change over time, and these changes can be accelerated through conversation. Canvassing on the doorstep for votes is commonly practised throughout the world. If my experience is anything to go by, being doorstepped by untrained enthusiasts of some particular political persuasion is very unlikely to change minds. However, there is another route to changing minds, and it shares something with the therapeutic engagement used in psychotherapy. A very successful path to changing someone's positions on topics such as marriage equality is 'deep canvassing',[18] where the canvasser attempts a conversation which is non-judgemental and involves active listening and careful and respectful exploration of the position of the canvassed person. Some research has shown that beliefs and attitudes can be changed by appeals that align with the views of the person being canvassed. But how do you know what values matter to the person? A field experiment was conducted by canvassers for Planned Parenthood of Northern New England, who listened to individual voters' moral values and then tailored their appeals to match.

These conversations had a significant impact on interest in taking political action and showed some evidence of changing policy attitudes. The method used was called 'personalized moral reframing' and involved interpersonal conversations like phone calls, workplace discussions or door-to-door canvassing. The conversations began with the canvasser asking for the voter's opinion and listening non-judgementally; this was followed by questions about experiences and emotions, and the sharing of personal stories. This approach is closer to a therapeutic conversation than to a typical political argument. It is very far from the standard political canvassing approach of the 'kick the bums out' (of office – 'vote for us, because we're better than them') and doorstep promises of 'what we will do for you and your neighbourhood'. To change minds, you must talk with respect and listen with care to what others have to say, and long-lasting, positive change in expressed prejudice and voting patterns becomes eminently attainable. This can be a really hard thing to do, and I am delighted it is something you can learn: I find I have a strong, almost automatic response of 'Oh, you can't believe that nonsense' when I occasionally have conversations with people repeating gibberish from their 'own research' – which often means being influenced by some blowhard on social media. They don't mean that they have deeply researched the relevant journals or interned in a molecular immunology lab.* Conversations do matter more than we know

---

* The things people believe that are empirically unfounded and empirically unmoored are almost without number. Here are a few of the more benign ones I have personally encountered: among gamblers, that certain numbers or sequences of numbers are lucky or unlucky; among foodies, that certain foods or substances have magical or healing properties ('food woo'); that you can predict the future by reading tea leaves or using cards, or some other form of divination (how come they're not all rich already?); that certain colours or shapes have special powers or meanings; that the world is controlled by a secret cabal of influential people (a cabal who don't seem to be very good at it, and whose identity varies depending on where you live, and the culture you grew up in); that crystals and stones have 'healing properties' – I find people from the west of Ireland less susceptible to this one, because of widespread knowledge of the local risks to health posed by accumulations of radon gas released by certain soils and stones (although this is most likely sampling bias on my part: https://gis.epa.ie/

or realise, for conversations can change cultures. But we have to know how this happens.

We – sometimes – disagree with each other during conversation. In fact, a certain amount of disagreement between people is a natural and, probably, necessary part of everyday life. Political parties, for example, routinely and publicly disagree with each other on policy prescriptions. This contest of ideas before the electorate might allow voters to make better and more informed choices than they might otherwise have done. (Of course, this assumes that the average voter is paying attention to the arguments, evaluating them and making a rational choice between the posed alternatives, a view that is probably not correct, for all sorts of reasons.)[19] Getting along with each other, despite even very strong disagreement, is a vital part of everyday cooperative life. Indeed, it is an essential life skill. We may all have larger goals that we share, despite disagreements about other goals; the larger goals may supersede, in some way, the smaller goals.

Michael Yeomans and his colleagues at Harvard Business School have explored 'conversational receptiveness'[20] – the idea that in conversation we can learn to listen to ideas we disagree with. They focus explicitly on training people to deal with viewpoints with which they may fervently disagree. Conducting a clever mix of experimental and field studies, they found that people rated by third-party evaluators as more receptive to counter-arguments – rather than rated by their own self-evaluations – were considered to be better teammates, advisers or workplace representatives. We are poor judges of how receptive other people think we are in conversation. This shouldn't be too surprising: as we have seen already, conversation is taxing, and making judgements

EPAMaps/Radon?&lid=EPA:RadonRiskMapofIreland). Of course, people sometimes believe things that are not so benign, but nature often finds a way to explain to them that these beliefs are not correct. Believing gravity is socially constructed, for example, is a grave error . . .

about what we think other people think of the quality of our listening is hard.

Yeomans and his colleagues explicitly focus on overcoming the unpleasant aspects of disagreement, by trying to understand how it might be possible to teach individuals how to deal with disagreement. They gathered participants who were presented with statements on controversial topics with which they disagreed. These might be statements such as 'The public reaction to recent confrontations between police and minority crime suspects has been overblown.' These participants were divided into two groups. One group was asked to write a response to statements where they indicated a willingness to listen to the position of the original author of that statement. To put it another way, half the participants were asked to express an openness to seeing the position of the other person in their written statements. The other participants responded with their own written statements but were not asked to indicate a willingness to listen to the contrary position. Yeomans and his colleagues ran the resulting essays through specially designed computer programs which picked out the elements of 'positive conversational receptivity' – the things that make you good at truly listening to, and truly hearing, what others have to say. Think of this as the equivalent of 'I hear what you're saying, and I'm willing to listen, and perhaps even change my mind because of it.' They also had human raters pick out what they judged as the elements of receptiveness during conversation, and compared these judgements to ones generated by a computer program designed to analyse the content of the conversations. They found the computer program performed relatively well at picking out these elements of conversational receptiveness.

In another phase of the work, they gathered pairs of government executives discussing controversial policy topics with partners who disagreed with their position on these topics. Here they asked participants to rate their sense of their own receptiveness to the arguments of others, finding that naive, untrained people are poor judges of how their own receptiveness is judged by others. We have privileged insider access only to our own thoughts about ourselves; we don't have this insider access to the thoughts others have about us – unless they tell us. How often does the silent but unexpressed thought that 'I'm a good listener' meet the silent, sarcastic rejoinder 'Yeah, you are?' We are often poor at judging how others see us, something known to poets down the ages. Robert Burns (1759–96), the Scottish poet, famously declaimed in his poem 'To a Louse': 'O wad some Pow'r the giftie gie us / To see oursels as ithers see us!'

Pushing the analysis of receptiveness further, Yeomans and his colleagues conducted a naturalistic field study of conversational threads from Wikipedia, using measures of conversational receptiveness. Wikipedia is a useful resource for studying receptiveness to contrary arguments, for it preserves the discussion threads behind consensual changes to the online text of individual Wikipedia entries. These discussions can sometimes be furious, but often they are careful discussions between individuals regarding the veracity or otherwise of claims made on Wikipedia. Remarkably, there are indeed markers of conversational receptiveness which could be picked out from these Wikipedia discussion threads. These markers were in turn useful predictors of the rapidity with which consensus could be reached about changes. If a Wikipedia editor or discussant displayed these markers of *truly listening* to the other person, then changes were more likely to be accepted.

'Naive' participants are people who are poor at understanding how others see their conversational receptiveness, and how they are perceived as hearing what the other person is saying. Is it possible to teach receptiveness? Can you teach people to listen more deeply, so that they try and hear what the other person is saying? And, importantly, can you teach them to provide explicit feedback demonstrating that they are hearing what is being said by the other person? The answer to all these questions seems to be 'yes' – you can be trained to be more receptive in conversation. An explicit recipe for receptiveness involves, during conversational flow, paying careful and specific attention to making positive statements rather than negations, explicitly acknowledging the other person's point of view, being willing to find points of agreement and, finally, using language to soften claims made during the conversation. Picking up on my own strong, almost automatic responses when listening to patent gibberish: my experience is that people very often do want to understand and are attempting to make some sort of sense of the world. Understanding what they are trying to say is hard, but can be worth it when you have a good-faith conversationalist. You can learn something new about how someone else sees the world.

*

'Investigative interviewing' is one of the names given to non-coercive methods of conducting conversations with sources – the victims, witnesses and suspects in cases being investigated by police in a legal or forensic context. Research into investigative interviewing shows there is a 'secret sauce' for gaining information: the secret sauce is 'rapport'. Rapport is a method of interviewing another person while displaying attentive interest to what they are saying, and a positive psychological disposition towards them. The interaction between the interviewer and the interviewee is made as respectful and as agreeable as possible in an attempt to foster a personal interaction, involving some form of empathic and meaningful human connection.

The components of rapport have been studied in detail by forensic psychologists, particularly in the context of attempts to elicit information from another person. Fiona Gabbert, a forensic psychologist at Goldsmiths, University of London, for example, has shown that the verbal components of rapport building are straight-forward:[21] you should use the person's name; disclose what you know, when appropriate, to the person that you're interviewing;

show interest in the person; listen actively; and offer empathic responses. The non-verbal components are, again, straightforward: being friendly; smiling; using body language that is open; making eye contact; and nodding at appropriate times during the conversation. And tone of voice is vitally important – speech must be sincere and respectful.

The investigative interview is more akin to a therapeutic encounter, using techniques clinical psychologists employ with a therapeutic client. This means that an interviewer can be trained in techniques that work, and they can undergo an apprenticeship. Because of video recordings, the components of interviewing that work and do not work can be discerned. A skilled forensic interviewer, on average, tends to be understanding of, comfortable with and sensitive to cultural differences; to be adept at placing individuals at ease; to have a good bedside manner; to have strong impulse control, being able to damp down their response to whatever it is that they are being told; to be capable of engaging in active listening; and to be able to understand and anticipate developments in their environment, particularly in high-stress or high-risk situations ('situational awareness').[22] And the key point is that these skills can be trained – they can be systematically taught to others.

These kinds of explicitly instructed and trained interventions changed the evaluation of the willingness to listen of the trained person compared to untrained individuals. The advice to 'Listen as hard as you can'[23] gives the space and opportunity to the other person to speak, and say what it is that they need to say on a particular topic. 'Listen as hard as you can' is difficult advice to follow, but if you want to be a good listener, then letting the other person speak, and explicitly framing the conversation as one within which they have the freedom to speak – without being contradicted – is the place to start. Conversation then becomes a 'safe place' in which to say what it is you truly think – something good psychotherapists have known for generations.

The key lesson here is that your capacity to truly listen to another person does not just depend on what they are saying; it also depends critically on you *as a listener*, and the conversational strategy you bring to bear. Going into a difficult conversation – indeed any conversation – where it is clear to the other person that you value the importance of active listening, rapport and offering respect is the way forward. Eschewing conversational gambits involving aggression, domination or status seeking will make the conversation more enjoyable for you and your interlocutor, and you will gain more information from the conversation than you might otherwise have done. This lesson occurs time and again – active listening, deliberately engaging in rapport and offering respect during conversations are as vital in domains as diverse as clinical interviewing for medical diagnostics, forensic interviewing for intelligence gathering and attempting to reconstruct a memory in social situation as they are in everyday life. Truly, try to 'listen as hard as you can'.

*

Let's deconstruct what is going on during a conversation, according to a simple rubric: there is a conversation occurring, so it must take place between two people; one person asks questions, and the other provides answers (thereby drawing upon their prior experiences – their memories – to answer the questions being asked). And the direction of the conversation alternates or flips: the questioner becomes the answerer; there is a back-and-forth. And during conversation we alternate phases of breathing: when I'm speaking, I'm breathing out, and you are breathing in; and when you speak, this reverses. In conversation, we describe and discuss all sorts of things: we might describe our bodily feelings (interoception), identifying where we might be feeling, or have been feeling, a pain. We might describe what we are, or have been, thinking (by introspecting – looking inward on our thoughts and describing them, which we will discuss in the next chapter). We might also describe what we think we are going to do (prospection). We might not be very good at any of these: we might misperceive our feelings and thoughts, and not recall them especially accurately. Nor might we recall the detail of our lives particularly well, because our memories fade in terms of detail, and all we are left with is the gist of the past. Nonetheless, we somehow make a success of it – we muddle through.

The language and memory systems of the brain are very closely locked together to enable you to have a conversation with another person. Language is central to human communication – this is obvious. But what role does memory play in communication? We will consider the uses of memories as they serve communication,[24] and we will especially try to understand how memory might fill out and enrich the conversations we have with other people. There are many potential ways to do studies on how memory serves and supports communication. In diary studies, for example, participants are asked to record the events of their everyday lives, and their memories are tested at some point afterwards to establish how much they remember and forget of their everyday lives.

Messages can be transmitted from one person to another – even to people from differing groups – but the accuracy of the message can be degraded as it passes from one person to another. There is a possibly apocryphal anecdote from the First World War, where an urgent message starts as 'Send reinforcements. We are going to advance,' gradually mutating through retelling up the line into 'Send three and fourpence. We are going to a dance.'[25] In a variation of this, psychologists have devised the 'serial reproduction paradigm' to study how messages are transmitted through chains of individuals. The serial reproduction paradigm is the fancy, technical name given to a systematised version of the well-known children's game, sometimes called 'Pass the Message' (other names include 'Telephone Operator', 'Grapevine' and 'Whisper Down the Lane'). One child writes down a message, then whispers the message to another child, who then seeks the next child to tell the message to, and this message is quietly retold through further ears and heads. The last child writes down what they have been told, and the starting and ending messages are compared, usually to much laughter, for the starting message and the final message might be dramatically and hilariously different.

Studies involving serial reproduction are, in principle, straight-forward to conduct. You start with a particular story, you tell it to one person, who in turn tells it to another person, who in turn tells it to another person. You record the story as it is being transmitted along the chain, and you can test what survives through its various reproductions. So, in summary, when we talk about the transmission of information between people, we're thinking about what gets shared, the ways people pass information around, and the fact that the information can morph into something else on the way.

What are the functions of such transmitted information? I argue here, as do others,[26] that conversational remembering is central to the creation of our shared social realities. Humans are a hypersocial species. We spend vast portions of our waking time thinking about our past interactions with others, or our future interactions with others. Our waking moments are filled with thoughts about who said what to whom, why what was said might have been said and what that means for us. Without this continual musing upon our social position relative to others, we would not be able to establish a shared social world. After all, we need to have common understandings about what we think is real. And conversation allows us to shape the positives and negatives of our shared worlds.

One ingenious investigation conducted a diary study in which participants recorded events in their daily lives. Participants were then asked which of these events in their daily lives they had discussed with others.[27] About two-thirds of the events recorded in the diary study had already been told to others *by the evening of the day that they occurred*. The point of such a study is that retelling stories inevitably draws on memory. What happens to the memories that are told to others? They might, rather like a virus, propagate or spread from the teller to the told – and then onwards to others again. A child might tell a parent a story, who in turn tells their spouse, who tells a sibling, and perhaps onwards again.

This broadcasting of experience recorded in memory is typical of human conversation. One study, for example, examined visits to a morgue by a medical class, and found that examinations of the contents of conversations by the students show they tell the story of the morgue visit far and wide.[28] On checking the thirty-three students involved in the visit to the morgue, they found that, within ten days, the students had told 881 people about their visit. In other words, there was a propagation rate (or R_0 as it called in epidemiology) – the speed at which the information was transmitted – through the social network of these students of a remarkable 26.7 for an interesting event in their lives. Findings like this support the idea that the personal need to share experiences – especially emotionally tinged experiences – with others gives rise to the rapid onward transmission of news. We naturally want to share our daily experiences, whether happy or dull, with others. We eagerly pass these stories on, sharing our emotions and experiences, our trials and tribulations. And as our stories circulate among other people, they evolve and change (like a game of 'Pass the Message'). We crave the connection and shared understanding that comes from sharing these stories, and others in turn feel the same urge, and can participate too.

Since the Covid pandemic we have become adept at discussing the so-called R-value, the reproduction rate of a virus. A reproduction rate above 1 means each person infected is infecting at least one other person. For memories retold through conversation, the retelling of memories has a reproduction rate vastly exceeding that for viruses (although conversations are probably more self-limiting than a virus like Covid – conversations probably only spread so far). Paralleling this finding, another study found about

58% of witnesses reported having discussed a witnessed incident with a co-witness to that incident.[29] We can't help it, can we? We talk to others about our memory of what we have seen, and this conversation shapes what we remember about what we have seen while also shaping the collective consensus about what we've seen. Here we arrive at one of the core ideas of this book – *a key function of our memories is intimately supporting social communication*.[30] Even though it feels as though our cognitive processes happen inside our head, it appears in some important senses that our social environment acts as an always-on stimulus for the emergence of our individual thoughts, ideas, dreams, reflections. In other words, our social world provides a kind of 'cognitive surface' on to which we project our busy mental lives, thereby allowing us to remember together in conversation.

*

We humans are, of course, complicated creatures with many needs and drives. One especially important drive is sense making. Humans are remarkable storytellers: we tell each other stories in conversation. Stories allow us to make sense of the world, and can serve the function of providing clues about identity and status within our world. This understanding in turn allows us to predict what is happening in our complicated social worlds. And the basis of this connectedness is, of course, our shared, constructed memories arising from the conversations we have with others throughout our lives. This has been eloquently described by the late and eminent British psychologist Sir Frederic Bartlett* as the 'effort after meaning':[31] our attempt – either by ourselves or in conversation with others – to impose a reliable understanding upon our world. And understandings vary between people. The Irish playwright George

---

* We will meet Bartlett again in subsequent chapters.

Bernard Shaw once noted that Britain and the US are 'two nations separated by a common language': a political conversation on liberalism between an American and a European will founder quickly, as the word 'liberal' has very different meanings in the two polities, while maintaining a particular meaning within each one.[32]

A new artistic movement arose in Paris in the late nineteenth century offering a new way of seeing the world – 'impressionism' (a phrase originally intended as an insult). Here, two critics bring different sensibilities to impressionist paintings, with one person seeing them as meaningless and the other seeing them as freeing and aesthetically powerful:

Critic 1: 'I hate these paintings; they look like random, unfinished daubs of colour, without meaning or purpose.'
Critic 2: 'You're coming at them from the wrong angle. These paintings allow you to see how light itself is captured so beautifully and dynamically. The ambiguity means you have to work a little at understanding the painting itself.'
Critic 1: 'But how is that beautiful? It just looks like a mess to me.'
Critic 2: 'You may not see the beauty in it, but I do. It's like saying a poem is meaningless because you don't understand it.'

(Critic 2 snickers to self, subvocally: 'Wait till you discover the interior monologue in these new-fangled novels . . .')

They're not quite at cross-purposes, but Critic 2 is explicit: you must make an effort in order to understand the meaning of these impressionist paintings: the 'effort after meaning'.

We can conclude that remembering in conversation is a 'social practice that promotes the formation of a collective memory'.[33] Remembering in conversation allows memories to form across a community (because we transmit our memories onwards to many others) which in time both reflects and shapes the identity of that community. Often, members of differing communities will ask themselves: 'How should we remember the events of our past? Should we remember them with shame? Should we remember them as humiliating? Or should we extol them as markers of our community's superior worth compared to others?'

Here, remembering in conversation can support or facilitate the creation of an identity-based, in-group/out-group membership. Just like our nations, these community memberships and community identities are *cognitively arbitrary*: they are not a feature of our social worlds, given to us from on high, as commandments inscribed on a tablet. There are lots of ways people try to define how you can be a member of a group or community – sometimes there is a crudely stated demand, based on 'blood'. This is ill-defined, but usually implies some familial relationship, or having two parents from the same place, meaning there is some form of imputed, connecting, genetic lineage.[34] The film *Goodfellas* offers a great example of this: two of the leads (played by the late Ray Liotta and by Robert de Niro, respectively) could not become 'made men' in the mafia, because they each had an Irish parent; but Joe Pesci's character could, because both his parents could be traced to Sicily – the 'old country'. A generation later, this requirement was seemingly dropped for American mafiosi; the rules for group membership can, and do, change over time, recognising new realities. And, of course, infidelities and other liaisons happen, and such lineages can only be truly determined because of late twentieth and early twenty-first century genomics; they are not given from on high.[35]

Others argue that some long-standing connection to a place – a parish, a town, a city, a region, going back through the ages – is necessary to be a member of a group; the gatekeeping to membership is based on memory. Communities are based on shared, and reshared, knowledge, favoured and exclusive access to that knowledge, shared rituals and a shared vision of the future, as well as an understanding of the past which includes some people but necessarily excludes others (we will discuss these ideas again in Chapter Eight, as foundational to the idea of nationhood). And, as we have seen, to have those thoughts you must have memories, and those memories impose a shape on your world, one that is mediated by words in conversation with others, and these views are only infrequently updated by data. These memories also facilitate mental time travel[36] – our remarkable mental ability to travel backwards and forwards mentally in time – back to a (perhaps) idealised past or forward to a blissful future, a land of 'milk and honey',[37] maybe.

When we talk to each other in conversation, especially if we are members of an oral culture or an oppressed society, what is it we are doing? What we are doing is preserving memories that would otherwise be forgotten or lost to us. Cultures with literacy and books benefit from the fast horizontal and vertical dissemination of knowledge – from older to younger, younger to older, younger to younger, older to older. Oral cultures differ – they preserve their histories in story and song – and the repository for these stories and songs is human memory. The very fact that differing groups, cultures and societies have differing origin stories – perhaps deriving from faulty or frail historical memories – means these origin stories are not all simultaneously correct. While the permanent loss of the record of a creation mythology can be decried as a broken bridge to a lost cultural past, because the culture that gave rise to it no longer exists, not believing in particular creation myths is not itself to be decried. Deliverance from false beliefs is as important as the attempt to discover, through empirical means, what is true.

Our individual memories foster common memories through the conversations we have with each other.[38] The very existence of this shared capacity is at the heart of our astounding and unique ability to create shared cultures that persist across time and space – our individual memory systems function as devices for sharing and exchanging ideas and information supporting the existence of those cultures through time. The ability to incorporate new information into these cultures, whether by individuals being born and dying, leading to a natural evolution of ideas, or by the movement of people into or out of societies, gives a capacity to those cultures to change and adapt over time.

In some respects, what I'm suggesting here seems almost trivial – that without an elaborate memory system in all our heads there would be no shared cultural memory repository. However, let's think about the counterfactual. I have discussed above Henry Molaison, the famous and most tested amnesic patient in history.[39] Henry was unable, for about fifty years, to participate meaningfully or effectively in the social, cultural or political life of his society, and had to live in a protected environment. During his mid- and late twentieth-century American life, there were numerous, momentous events, such as the assassinations of John F. Kennedy and Martin Luther King, the Vietnam War, the Civil Rights marches, the election of presidents and dramatic shifts in popular culture (particularly in movies, music and writing).

Henry was oblivious to these changes, though they formed the backdrop to daily life, identity formation and collective memory for Americans for decades, and still do. And this obliviousness was because Henry was amnesic – but that's not the whole of it. Let's work through the individual, social and cultural consequences of his amnesia: he was unable to participate in the shared conversations we have allowing information transmission within society. A conversation with him about Rosa Parks or John F. Kennedy would have been pointless, for they happened upon the scene after his 'frankly experimental' operation. He could not remember the identities of individual persons from one day to the next, even of people that he met regularly. This points to the heart of the tragedy of Henry's life: he was unable to bring to bear, during conversation, a regularly updated (and conversationally update-able) memory to facilitate conversational flow, with its use of imagination, construction of shared realities and reimagined futures, and thereby participate in everyday life and the changes occurring in popular culture.

Now, imagine a society entirely populated by individuals with amnesia like that suffered by Henry, with every day 'alone in itself'. This seems almost unthinkable, doesn't it? In such a society, nobody remembers anything, so nobody learns anything. Nobody knows who anyone else is from day to day; in fact, this widespread loss of memory ensures that it's not really a society in any mean-ingful way. Everyone has to start over every time they meet, as if they have never met before. The contents of the conversations people have with each other are lost, and lost for ever – the con-versations they have are not encoded in the memory systems of the brains of any of the conversing individuals. A society without memory has no capacity to repair itself; it has no capacity to evolve; it has no capacity to adapt; it has no capacity to remember or to learn.

By contrast, the world we live in is not one populated by amnesiacs (although our unwillingness to learn from the past occasionally makes it feel like we do!). The crux of our social and collective lives involves an overlooked miracle, one that is so close to us that we find it difficult to see it: namely, our ability to remem-ber things quickly and effectively, to report on our thoughts and feelings, to shape what we are saying quickly to the conversation we are having with other people. *Without our memories, no culture is possible, and society is lost.* If there is no memory of the past, who is to say what the present is?

If nothing extends beyond the present moment, who is to say what the future will be? With dementia, our ability to imagine something beyond ourselves, a future timeline for ourselves or our society at large, is lost, and lost for ever. Yet our societies survive the loss of individuals and the loss of the memories of individuals, contriving to continue their existence through conversation – recycling and retelling memories between us all, ensuring our society is preserved – and not dependent on the memories present in any one particular individual's head. Before we discuss how this is possible, we do need to have some understanding of the conversations we have with ourselves – or at least of what comes and goes through our minds as we think about the world and our place in it – and this is where we will turn next.

2.
THE BUZZ OF MENTAL LIFE: THE CONVERSATIONS WITHIN US

I'm sure you're aware of the buzz of your mental life: the thoughts, images, notions, feelings, confusions, anxieties, attention grabs, diversions, ear-worms and all the rest of it. You puzzle about something said to you; you think about hunger pangs and lunch; about how to escape the droner in front of you. And so much more. Descartes famously said, 'Cogito, ergo sum': I think, therefore I am. A deeper question is how it is possible for the kilo and a half (more or less) of organic matter comprising your brain to have a mental life, to be aware of its own existence – a question (still) awaiting an answer. More tractable, though, is asking about the components of your mental life, and how they come to be, and how they relate to each other – what your ongoing thoughts, feelings, anxieties, delights and all that jazz comprise in the course of your daily life. Psychology has attempted to answer that question for over one hundred years, and answers are starting to come into view. Just as spectacularly, we're starting to understand the underlying brain networks that give rise to differing aspects of mental life.

Let's begin by going back to the dawn of psychology as a scientific discipline as it attempted to understand our mental processes.[1] Historically, the route to understanding our mental processes was through introspection – describing as best you can what is going through your head at this moment. Or it might be what was going through your head (as best you can remember it) at some previous point in time – maybe reflecting on a past conversation, realising that you were feeling anxious during the conversation and that this might have affected how you interacted with the other person. Or it could even be anticipating what might go through your head at some future time – perhaps thinking about an upcoming meeting and anticipating feeling nervous about speaking in public. Then you must try to put into words what you are thinking and feeling.

Introspection – *looking inward on our mental lives as observers* – was introduced into experimental psychology by Wilhelm Wundt (1832–1920), who in Leipzig in 1879 founded the first ever psychological laboratory. Wundt was an exacting scientist who wanted to train introspectionists to be objective observers of their own thoughts and feelings, which they were expected to describe to the experimenter. Wundt would engage a subject in an experimental task (e.g. colour naming, recollecting some significant event from the past, reading particular passages of prose, counting objects). He required his participants to act as observers of their own mental lives, writing (a little opaquely to modern eyes) that 'the Introspectionist must, as far as possible, grasp the phenomenon in a state of strained attention and follow its course'.[2]

This is a very demanding form of inspection of one's own inner mental life: you have to 'grasp' what is happening in your own consciousness as you pay attention to something – say, a sound, a flickering light or a scene or conversation of some sort – and then find the words to describe what you grasp. Such demands find a modern-day echo in the injunction to engage in 'mindfulness' – to observe, without judgement, the stream of thoughts and feelings wandering and coursing through your consciousness. Nowadays, in an experimental psychology lab, we would probably say something like: 'You're presently seated in the dark in front of a computer monitor. I want you to pay close attention to the computer screen, and when you see the faint triangle, press the button as fast as possible; if you see anything else (such as a faint square), you should do nothing.' Or we might conduct the same procedure, but while you're lying on your back in a brain scanner to try to figure out what might be going on in your brain while performing this task. Modern brain scanners are well adapted to this kind of task, able to present visual stimuli, as well as sounds played through headphones (or even electric shocks, if you are studying pain). You can even watch movies in a brain scanner, if you're so inclined – and, as we will see later, this is useful if you want to understand the response of the brain to coherent, extended stories.

In effect, Wundt was asking his participants to repeatedly throw a bucket into the 'stream of consciousness' (a phrase introduced by the psychologist William James in 1890). By describing the contents of the successive buckets, we might thereby build a picture of our mental lives. Introspection was also much discussed by James, who described it as 'the looking into our own minds and reporting what we there discover'. Introspection even forms the core of certain types of psychotherapy, where the client is encouraged to talk, at length, about their feelings, thoughts, memories and the like. Introspectionist psychology also had a marked, if indirect, influence on the development of the novel in the early twentieth century, when storytelling became centred on the 'interior monologue' – the description of the thoughts passing through the protagonist's mind. (William James was the brother of the novelist Henry James, famous for his early use of the interior monologue and stream of consciousness in his novels.)[3]

Some parodied introspection: knowing our capacity for

self-delusion, the American short-story writer Ambrose Bierce (of *The Devil's Dictionary* fame) wrote in his *Epigrams of a Cynic* (1912) that the 'most charming view in the world is obtained by introspection', thereby hinting at the delusions and lack of self-knowledge that might accompany the attempt to look inward at our own mental lives. Experimental psychology started with introspection as its method of choice, but over time it fell into disfavour, replaced by behaviourism and approaches focused on observable behaviour. Introspection never disappeared as a method within psychology, however – it was renamed 'self-reporting', and self-report tests have become the core of personality psychology and social psychology, as well as many other disciplines (such as political science and marketing).

Much effort has been devoted to constructing reliable and valid scales and questionnaires to measure, for example, personality, or the depth and extent of major depressive disorder, and the like. Scales and questionnaires are deployed in clinics and other settings throughout the world to assist in the making of clinical diagnoses. And all these scales more or less rely on respondents providing answers to questions, offering ratings of how they have felt, what they have done and so on. These scales are often used to assist during other forms of clinical investigation – from X-ray and other scans to biopsies – which might be uninterpretable without them. The interpretation of a shadow on the lungs detected by X-ray depends in part on the honesty of the person disclosing if they smoke, how much and for how long. Disclosing that you were (or are) a smoker – as opposed to reporting having been exposed to asbestos – will help the radiographer or radiologist make sense of the images of the lungs they have to interpret.

These differing kinds of self-disclosures require you to provide answers by interrogating your own memory. The interviewer does not have direct access to your memories – only you have that. We are generally fluent and fluid at providing such responses, and we expect each other to be able to provide such answers quickly and reliably. Claiming that you can't remember will often be met with disbelief, unless you have (verifiable) blackouts, amnesia or some such condition. However, the memory systems of the brain are not well designed to provide the precise answers we may sometimes be called upon to give – little wonder the answers we give to questionnaires and scales can (and do) mislead ourselves and others. We are often very poor at the high-precision recall of information, even if it was information you used for a considerable period of time. If you work at an organisation requiring you to change your password every couple of months, ask yourself 'What was my third-to-last password?' I'm sure you'll flunk this just as quickly and easily as I have (just) done. Or try to recall pi to seven or eight decimal places . . .

Modern technology allows us, with a speed and precision that would have astounded Wundt, to see what might be happening in the brain when we talk about ourselves. We can now peer into the brain while people perform memory tasks. You might be invited to learn a list of word pairs on a computer screen. These word pairs might be, for example: apple–pear, plum–peach, orange–banana, book–paper, car–wheel, phone–mouse and so on. Then you are presented with the first word of the pair and must recall the second word, and so on through the list. Your brain can be imaged while you are performing this task, and activity during learning or recall of the words can be compared to a suitable control task. In principle, these kinds of experiments allow you to figure out the contribution of certain brain networks to particular tasks. The consistent activation of a particular brain region during a memory task, for example, provides important clues to the possible involvement of that brain region in the neural processes supporting memory. The 'turning on' of the hippocampal formation during a memory task is an important clue that it is involved in memory; loss of memory after hippocampal damage gives another important clue. Gradually, you can start to construct a case that this particular structure (the hippocampal formation) must have an important role in memory.

The neuropsychological processes here are complicated. You must first read the words (and reading means you've spent a considerable period *learning* how to read): the word image must pass via the eyes to various way stations in the visual parts of the brain, where it is decoded and turned into sound. The words also pass through brain networks for memory, where a search is performed for the missing word of the pair, and then the word pair is completed. Next, the word pair must pass through brain regions concerned with articulating and making sounds, and then you must speak words and sentences. And then you find out if you are correct in your recall or not. The early part of reading and recall happens below the level of consciousness, and only the results of the search enter into consciousness and are then articulated.[4] Typically, the brain delivers these answers in well under a second (as measured using electrodes implanted in the brain for certain types of neurosurgery). You only become conscious of the word pair after about one-third to one-half of a second or so, and then you report this to the psychologist as part of the test.[5]

There is another method of discovering what we are thinking, feeling and doing at any given moment: it is called 'experience sampling'. Experience sampling generally involves using modern technology, such as smartphone apps. Think of it as a form of instant introspection: an app pings you randomly during the day and asks you to give quick ratings of what you are thinking, feeling, doing, seeing, hearing at that moment. The reality is that we are very poor at recalling what we were thinking, feeling and doing at particular points in time. Can you recall how happy you were at 2 p.m. last Tuesday? Or the Wednesday before that? Don't fool yourself. You can't. You need to take contemporaneous records.

During experience sampling, you might rate your happiness on a scale of 1–10 every hour for several days or more; or keep a journal and write down your thoughts and feelings every time you hear a specific trigger word or phrase, such as 'stress' or 'anxiety'. You might use a smartphone app to take a photo of your current environment and rate your level of contentment when pinged. Or you might wear a wristband that tracks heart rate, sleep and physical activity, and give mood ratings every waking hour. You might participate in a mindfulness meditation session, and be pinged to rate your level of focus and clarity for some period of time afterwards. The possibilities are numerous, and constrained only by experimenter ingenuity and technological limitations.

As we shall see, experience sampling gives us an unprecedented picture of the moment-to-moment contents of consciousness – to capture what is going on in people's heads. In the initial versions of experience sampling pioneered by the late Hungarian-American psychologist Mihaly Csikszentmihalyi, participants were provided with bleepers and, when bleeped, wrote down in diaries what they had just been thinking about. This is experience sampling of introspection on the fly, when you are out and about in the world. And this technique can be readily adapted to the data-harvesting techniques used by mobile phone apps that we have become so familiar with – mobile data collection can be used to validate or test what people say they have been doing.

In an interesting example of this method, the renowned social psychologist Roy Baumeister and his colleagues examined the contents of the mental lives of people going about their everyday business.[6] In particular, they wanted to test the idea that people think more about the future than about the past. They recruited a sample of 200 people; these participants were pinged via SMS text message six times per day between 9 a.m. and 9 p.m. They were asked to indicate their emotional state on a scale of –3 (very sad) to +3 (very happy), and their state of physiological arousal from –3 (very relaxed) to +3 (very excited). Participants, when pinged, were also asked whether they were thinking about the past (defined as more than five minutes ago); the present, defined as the things that have happened within the current five-minute time window; or the future (defined as more than five minutes hence). They were also then asked to indicate the time window: was it today, tomorrow or further away in time? They captured about 6,700 mobile samples regarding the reported contents of their participants' thoughts. Thinking about the here and now comprised about 53% of thoughts reported, whereas thinking exclusively about the past made up a minority of thoughts (about 5% or so of thoughts reported) and thinking about the future comprised about 24% of thoughts. Thus we are often preoccupied by the here and now (unsurprisingly, for we must live in the present), but devote a lot of our thinking time to the future – about a quarter of our thoughts).

These apps provide a picture of the active mind *in the moment* – they provide a readout of your current experience. This is not the same as the evaluation you might subsequently make of that experience; but remember, the experience you have had and the memory of the experience you have had are not the same things. Imagine being taken for a long drive in a car as a passenger. You sit there, whizzing along the motorway, gazing out of the window, occasionally listening to the radio or chatting to the driver, and you do this for perhaps two or three hours. If you were asked during the journey what you were thinking about, you might report some mild boredom or mind blankness, or the like. And then you arrive at your destination, step out of the car, get your bags and say hello to the people at your destination. And little trace of the journey remains in your memory, unless something unusual has happened. Or let's say you holidayed at a beach resort where you had a great time relaxing on the beach, sea swimming and trying new foods. However, on returning home and reflecting on the trip, you might find yourself focusing more on the long flight or the crowded hotel: the experience of being on holiday and the memory of the holiday are not the same thing. The experience is what is happening in the moment, whereas the memory is a simplified, schematised version of the experience, one influenced by your emotions, your conversations afterwards with family and friends, your biases and time passing.

Now, cast your mind back and try to remember the fine details of your trip: you've just experienced the car journey, but you remember little specifically of it. This is the paradox at the core of our mental lives: what we remember of what we experience and what we have experienced often differ considerably. As the psychologist Daniel Kahneman expresses it: 'I am my remembering self, and the experiencing self, who does my living, is like a stranger to me.'[7] The writer Oliver Burkeman elaborates another version of this paradox: 'We tend to remember having been happy in the past much more frequently than we are conscious of being happy in the present.'[8] Both of these statements are very telling – we live in a more abstracted way than we are ever conscious of doing, mentally moving backwards and forwards through, and then recentring ourselves into the present moment.

*

We have all had the experience of our minds wandering off topic while we are attempting to pay attention to a boring task. Mind wandering can be dangerous if you allow your mind to drift too much while performing certain tasks; if you allow your mind to wander while driving, you may cause a fatal collision. Letting your mind drift in a classroom is less fatal: the penalty for mind wandering might be receiving some (perhaps misconceived) invective from your teacher. We flicker between zooming in on particular tasks and zooming out, perhaps while considering the larger picture of our lives. A key conclusion of modern psychological science is that mind wandering is characteristic of thought. It shouldn't be considered a design defect of the functioning of our brains. Mind wandering can be deleterious for tasks requiring continuous concentration, but it can equally facilitate tasks requiring creativity and problem solving:[9] for an artist, mind wandering can be deleterious for tasks requiring continuous concentration, such as rendering a detailed portrait or a very exacting still-life painting. Attention to fine and particular details, accurately rendered, would suffer if the artist's mind wanders off, leading to errors and mistakes in the final piece.

However, mind wandering can facilitate tasks requiring creativity and problem solving, such as conceptualising a new piece of art or coming up with a unique composition, through the accidental collision of ideas and visual images. Similarly, in computer programming, mind wandering can be deleterious for tasks requiring continuous concentration such as debugging complex code or writing low-level system software, whereas mind wandering can facilitate tasks requiring creativity and problem solving such as designing a new software architecture, app or algorithm.

How does the brain support the complex mental states associated with mind wandering and with focusing on particular tasks? In an elegant study, the neuroscientist Hao-Ting Wang and her colleagues at the University of York in the UK conducted a large-scale study in which they recruited 165 participants to try to understand the composition of everyday mental experience.[10] Their special focus was the disparateness of thought generated by the wandering mind during everyday life. Their hardy participants were studied over a period of several weeks: their brains were imaged while they performed a variety of tasks; they filled in (self-report) questionnaires sampling psychological functioning; and records were taken of their moments of mind wandering. These elements of the study focus on everyday conscious experience: the extent to which our thoughts and memories are present-oriented, as well as future-oriented; and whether our thoughts and memories are principally concerned with negotiating our social status, our social position within groups or our cooperative lives with each other.

Indeed, to delve deeper here, the larger question is the extent to which our thoughts and memories serve to construct the nature of the reality we form together. Imagine a group of people who have experienced a traumatic event, such as a war, who share their stories and memories with each other in a conversation. Their understanding of the event is shaped by the individual thoughts and memories they share in the conversation. As the conversation progresses, the shared understanding of the event becomes more detailed and nuanced as they construct an overall memory of the event. Individual thoughts and memories serve as the building blocks for constructing the shared reality of the group through conversation. The group's collective understanding is shaped by the individual thoughts and memories shared and, in turn, these collective understandings shape reality for the group.

The study conducted by Wang and colleagues is necessarily complex, for it requires participants to be willing to undergo repeated brain scanning, as well as to (repeatedly) complete other tests relating to their thoughts and feelings. Sometimes the tasks the participants undertake seem a little dull: they might have to compare shapes and colours with other shapes and colours, and decide if they are similar or different. You get visual-search and pattern-matching challenges like this all the time in a supermarket: go to the dental-care aisle and try to pick out your favourite toothpaste from the many varieties on offer, or try to find your favourite jam among the hundreds on offer in the preserves aisle. Ask yourself – how hard are you concentrating while doing this mundane chore? The experimental task simulates aspects of these kinds of chores in everyday life, where you are perhaps paying no more than partial attention. During these 'dull' tasks, participants are occasionally interrupted and asked, via the computer, if their mind is on the task (wholly, partially or not at all) or if their mind is wandering away from the task. They are probed about the kinds of thoughts they are having: whether they are present-oriented or future-oriented, or if they are thinking about themselves or about others, or about their own emotions, and whether the content of their thoughts is in the form of images or words.

By bringing together into a single register (via advanced data-analysis techniques) brain imaging, experience sampling and participants' self-reports of their own past states, Hao-Ting Wang and her colleagues built a comprehensive picture of the contents of thinking and of mind wandering. Overall, they found that mind wandering is 'heterogeneous' – that it consisted of mixed, assorted, diverse thoughts. This was to be expected. The contents of mind wandering in one person, given differences in traits, experience and memory, are of course going to be different from the specific contents of mind wandering in another person. But, more interestingly, different types of mind wandering were associated with different types of psychological functions in differing individuals, with the key finding of a strong link between mind wandering and individual creativity.

This very elegantly conducted group of studies suggests memory, creativity and spontaneous thought are strongly related to each other. To spell this out a bit: when writing a short story, a person may draw on specific memories of a trip they took to a beach as a child. These memories may spark a creative idea for a scene in their story where the main character also goes to a beach and experiences something significant. Musing further – spontaneous, wandering, thought – leads them to develop the details of this scene (such as particular emotions the character feels, the imagery of the setting), all through using memories of their own childhood trip as inspiration.

Default mode activity is strongly associated with both forward and backward mental time travel. The natural assumption would be that the contents of our thinking would be biased towards the past, but it seems we spend the bulk of our waking life thinking about the present and the future.[11] The central paradox emerging from these studies is that although we might think memory is about remembering the past, in fact our memory serves our present and future adaptive needs. That is not to say that memories of the past are not recalled – of course they are – but they are recalled usually in the service and context of ongoing behavioural and cognitive and social needs. Moreover, the brain networks that think about the past are also much the same brain networks that allow us to think about the future. That memory you have of glorious summer days infuses imagined future holidays on a Tuscan hillside. That continuing horror you have of a beach holiday is contaminated by the windswept, rain-damp, caravan holidays of your childhood. The remembered and reconstructed past, the imagined and longed-for holiday, all arrive in a confluence in the present moment, driving your thoughts and changing the direction of how you think you might be spending your future time.

*

Reporting our 'instantaneous' thoughts and feelings – even if these are about the past or future – is one thing. But our mental lives are much richer than can be revealed by instantaneous reports of what we are currently thinking about. We have, as individuals, a strong, narrative, autobiographical sense of ourselves. Indeed, we love to read the biographies, memoirs and autobiographies of others, and to listen to and watch interviews and chat shows where we can learn about the lives of others as they tell stories about themselves. We are also delighted to be offered the chance to tell our own stories, and we find it intrinsically rewarding when we do – that is, the brain's reward system is strongly activated when we get the chance to talk about ourselves![12] This rewarding effect of recalling happy, positive memories of our personal past life is so strong that it actively counters or reduces the effects of deliberately imposed laboratory stressors, such as having one's hand immersed in ice-cold water.[13] When tested, in conversation or in writing, we can quickly and easily offer a 'blurb' about our past life. We can tell our life story – we can pick out what we see as the important and formative events of our lives; in short, we can 'narrate' the story of our lives, and thereby impose order and meaning on our lives over time. This narrative is, of course, generated by our memories – we must select, pick, choose the elements of our past experience that are important to us, that have made us, in our own eyes, who we are.

Christin Köber and Tilmann Habermas, psychologists at the Goethe University in Frankfurt, were keen to understand how stable, in memory, are the details of our personal past – our own autobiography.[14] They conducted a longitudinal study over eight years of autobiographical memories and of personal life stories (or 'narratives'), tracking each participant individually over time to investigate the stability of their memories. Participants were asked to recall their seven most important memories. Additionally, they were asked to provide a narrative account of their autobiography – their life story for the life they had lived to this point. These kinds of studies allow an investigation into the relative importance to a person's own personal autobiography of the events of their lives at differing times.

An event looming large in your memory at the age of eight – one which seems very important at that age – might have disappeared from memory by age twelve, for example. A child of eight, for instance, might decide that their most important memory was of the wonderful present that they received at their last birthday, but by twelve this memory of the wonderful present has disappeared. Thus a first important question is discovering how stable are the selected memories of people in terms of assessing their importance over time: do the details drift over time, or are they reliably recalled at differing time points? A second question is how stable our life stories are over time; they might remain relatively stable, or they might change from time to time, or they might show change at one point in life and less change at other points. As is well known, both ageing and maturation can affect memory too. So Köber and Habermas also investigated how age affects these two aspects of normal human memory function.

Having access to your own personal autobiographical narrative and the general facts of your life, recorded at differing time points, allows an examination of how these two aspects of memory are coupled – or not. Repeated testing of narrative memory over time allows you to determine how stable memories are, and how much change happens in memory. It also allows you to

examine the changes in how you narrate your own autobiographical story over time. This is a very rich way of directly addressing
questions to do with how the stories we tell ourselves change over
time and how these are, in turn, affected by the memories we
believe are most important.

During the period of most rapid personal development – that
is, the younger years of life through to the middle or slightly later
adolescent period – what counts as an important memory for an
individual changes quite considerably. By contrast, life stories
showed an increase in stability with age and, perhaps not unex-
pectedly, a greater coherence in the life narrative. What we think
of as significant and important memories may bear little relation
to our life story. For example, we might regard our first day at
school as a very important memory – perhaps at the age of eight,
perhaps even at the age of twelve – but by age sixteen the memory
of the first day at school might be salient (but not especially
important). Köber and Habermas also found an interesting bifur-
cation in the stability of memory. The most important memories
decreased in stability as the time intervals between the memories
grew, and showed an increase in stability with age only from late
adolescence to late adulthood. To put it another way, memories
chosen as most important by the younger children decreased in
importance over time, unlike the memories chosen by the older
participants. As we get older, we get better at imposing a story
upon our own life's trajectory that *we find* coherent. An important
paradox therefore emerges. When comparing the stability of the
seven most important memories to life narratives, important
memories are more stable when you are younger but become less
stable as you get older, whereas your life story becomes more
stable when you are older (from sixteen years and beyond).

We spend a substantial fraction of our mental lives (perhaps
40% of our waking time) thinking and musing about the big picture of our lives. Focusing on the larger picture might be a more
efficient way for us to recall important components of our past and

place ourselves on a trajectory through time. We are deeply concerned with thoughts about the future. To reflect a constant theme of this book, we engage in substantial amounts of mental time travel, effortlessly whizzing forward in time, thinking about what might be at some point in the future. We revise and rework our 'narrative selves' over time: our narrative self is like a Wikipedia page – it is largely stable, and may seem much the same each time we check it out, but it is in fact continuously and subtly revised. In this way, we incorporate new elements into our personal identity, while discarding or de-emphasising other elements, in the service of keeping a narrative sense of self. This is known as 'self-referential thought' – our wandering minds focus on information about ourselves and our position and status within our social worlds. In turn, this allows us to determine our long-term goals, by going on 'journeys of the mind' into the past, present and future – the everyday magic of mental time travel.[15]

*

We now have hints of the brain structures involved in this form of mind wandering. The neuropsychologist Cornelia McCormick and her colleagues at University College London have examined mind wandering in patients with selective damage to the hippocampal formation – and who have a dense amnesia (similar to Henry Molaison's).[16] Their study is so ingenious that light is thrown on the remarkable phenomenon of 'mind blanking' – where we are not thinking about anything at all and our minds are seemingly devoid of thought at the moment when tested.

Many studies have now shown that prominent features of mind wandering include visuospatial images as well as mental time travel. Moreover, we tend to think in scenes and images when focusing on our past, present and future.[17] McCormick and her colleagues studied a group of six patients with selective damage to the hippocampus on both sides of the brain, accompanied by memory impairment – a very rare type of patient indeed. The selectivity of the damage they had suffered could be seen using modern brain-imaging techniques. These patients were, on average, fifty-seven years old, and about seven years before had suffered hippocampal damage from a rare and selective infection of the brain. As with Henry Molaison, these patients had normal working memory and could keep in mind the instructions for the tasks they were given long enough to complete them. McCormick and her colleagues had research assistants shadow the hippocampal patients during a day-long visit to the lab. While testing the patients over the course of the day, the research assistants would regularly ask the patients what was on their minds in the moments prior to being asked. Asking the patients multiple times over the course of a structured set of days, combined with brain scanning, psychological testing, breaks, lunches, periods of relaxation and the like, allows you to get good samples of what these patients might be thinking about at particular moments.[18]

What might be the logical outcomes of these 'thought' probes? There are at least the following options: you might be engaged in mind wandering in relation to what you are currently experiencing ('perceptually coupled' mind wandering); you might be thinking about something else entirely ('perceptually decoupled' mind wandering); or you might be thinking about nothing at all ('mind blanking'). Other possibilities for testing would include asking for your thoughts about where you are positioned in time: you might be wondering about the past, present or future, for example. Equally, you might be thinking about something very specific in terms of knowledge about the world (such as the shape of the switch on the kettle that you are about to make a cup of tea with). Or you might be engaged in episodic thinking, where your thoughts combine time, place and a feeling of re-experiencing the past, or even anticipating the future (avoiding the caravan park holiday, and calculating how to make the Tuscan flight instead). The final step is coding the thought as verbal or visual.

When probed, the patients did not report mind blanking, but did show decreased mental time travel; their mental time travel was less rich, and was marked by the absence of visual scenes when thinking – seemingly these patients have mostly verbal thoughts. One important conclusion is that hippocampal patients with episodic memory loss (they are amnesic) do show at least some mind wandering. The selective hippocampal damage these patients have has a huge effect on the content of the mind wandering they engage in. Healthy participants thought about the past, the present and the future, and did so in visually rich scenes, where they could see, in their mind's eye, a view of the events they were thinking about. By contrast, the patients typically mind wandered around topics mostly related to the present, and did not spend much time mind wandering back to the past or forward to the future.

Key components of how we think about the past, the present and the future involve vivid and rich details, including visual scenes. We go on a 'journey of the mind', taking us away from the demands of the immediate present. We go on this mind journey using rich visual scenes, which requires an intact memory system if we are to generate these thoughts and scenes at all. We can conclude with reasonable certainty that a particular structure in the brain – the hippocampal formation – enables us, because of its key role in memory, to deepen and substantially enrich the contents of our mind wandering and thus of our imaginings.

We do not yet know if hippocampal damage impoverishes our narrative life stories. Given the key role the hippocampal formation plays in supporting the fine detail of our mind wandering, providing rich visuospatial scenes, layering in memories from the past, it seems reasonable to suggest that the hippocampal function would play a central role in narrative life-story creation. The memories we are discussing here are necessarily those of the individual person. But many memories of the individual are social or are of life events that have occurred in a social context – a conversation, a party or a sporting event (such as a football match). Others again are of major and minor historical events, but these shape the thoughts, memories and feelings of the individuals within the nation. Trying to understand the relations between individual memory and collective memory is what we will next explore.

3.

SOLVING PROBLEMS TOGETHER: BEES DO IT, THE BORG DO IT AND WE DO IT TOO

Suppose you like to drive your car to work, because you think it will be a speedy way to get there, but you find everyone drives their cars to work also, and you are inevitably slowed down by all those other cars. To every car driver, every other car is traffic. There are lots of ways to try and solve this problem: building more roads is one;[1] providing ample and frequent public transport is another. To build roads or provide more public transport requires collective action: financing, land purchases, design, tendering and lots more besides. This type of problem is known as a 'collective action' problem – which arises when outcomes are worse if no one works together and better if everyone works together in a coalition of some sort for a period of time. Problems of collective action arise in situations where each person would benefit if everyone cooperated, but for differing reasons individuals may fail to cooperate.[2] Solving some vital coordination problem for a group is how what might be very loosely called a 'collective mind' might arise (although it isn't a mind in any meaningful sense: it is a means of aggregating a series of individual voices to generate an outcome for everyone). A 'coordinating authority' of some sort is required to make things happen.

We solve collective coordination and action very often through conversation, story and narrative, which are 'the main engines for synchronisation of individually held memories'.[3] This is a big claim, but not an entirely surprising one,[4] for our conversations and interactions with each other are how we regularly replenish and update our individual memories, allowing us to mentally time travel and imagine afresh. We humans have devised other remarkable mechanisms to solve coordination problems. We use markets and pricing mechanisms to deal with allocation and distribution problems (and markets rely on the shared cognitive realities of mutually binding contracts and enforcement mechanisms). We also use deliberative and consultative means (legislative assemblies or executive boards of organisations, for example) and decision-making systems (including voting) to arrive at collective decisions (with conversation at the heart of deliberation). We humans also coordinate our behaviour via shared language and conversation (in small groups), or via cognitive artefacts such as poems, songs, newspapers, books and social media (for larger groups).

The vast collective shared entities where most of us live and die – our cities – must, and do, solve collective-action problems on a grand scale in order for our cities to exist at all. The largest city in the world is the Tokyo Metropolitan Area, with a population of about 37.5 million people, living together with crime rates that are among the lowest in the world. About 40 million people use the Tokyo public transport system every day.[5] And they do so largely without incident – an astonishing achievement of infrastructure, timetabling and humans' trust in each other.

Other organisms have collective-action problems too. Social

insects are creatures such as termites, honeybees and ants; these species build, maintain and defend elaborate nests serving the collective, rather than the individual, good. Not all insects, of course, are social. Many meet only for the purposes of reproduction and then go their own way. Insect colonies are complex, making use of different types of labour, including resource gathering (particularly food), but defence of the colony and repair of the nest are also paramount. These nests and hives bear more than a passing resemblance to our cities: with specialised labour, means of communication, construction and trafficking with the world beyond the nest. The collective-action problem has been studied intensely in social insects. These social insects solve this problem in a variety of ways, perhaps by using chemical signals (called 'social pheromones') to coordinate behaviour.

Researchers who examine collective behaviour in these insect colonies refer to these creatures as having a 'social physiology'.[6] The processes within their bodies are attuned to, and have evolved to respond to, signals within the social network important for sustaining the colony. Hormonal signals and pheromones are particularly important, but other forms of signalling such as social dancing and distress signals are also used. Pheromones and hormones prompt certain types of behaviour. Foraging for food, for example, is driven not by the hunger of the foragers, but instead by pheromonal signals from the larvae needing food. Thus a complicated insect colony can be sustained over many generations by coordinating the behaviour of the individuals within it via a variety of special signals.

A different vision for coordinating collective behaviour appears in the *Star Trek* science-fiction television and movie series, where cybernetic humanoids known as 'the Borg' represent a grave and mortal threat to many other (though not all) alien species. The Borg 'assimilate' captured individuals into the 'Collective', where each individual, known as a drone, is connected to a sophisticated 'group mind' or 'hive mind', allowing the drones to quickly share the same thoughts and learn new things. In confrontations, the Borg speak collectively, saying that 'Resistance is futile' and bluntly asserting 'You will be assimilated.' The mind of the Borg is collective, producing instant coordination of thought and behaviour among all the drones connected to a network. Personality and individuality are all lost – only the Borg Collective is immortal.

The coordination problem is solved by plugging each drone into a network that connects all drones together. It is unclear how the network itself makes decisions, particularly decisions of great importance. In some versions of the Borg, a Borg queen either speaks for or decides on behalf of or mediates between the collective inputs of all the drones. It may be that some form of pattern matching against memory is performed, and thereby a problem solved, based on what has been learned from those species previously assimilated by the Borg.

These two cases – actual social insects, imagined alien beings – represent part of the spectrum of possibilities for solving coordination problems. Humans have solved the problem in a different way, by means of conversation and discussion. We solve it by using formal and informal deliberative assemblies of some sort – a universal feature of small- and large-scale human life: we have meetings, boards, parliaments, fora, legislative assemblies, citizen's assemblies, town halls, gatherings. Some are very old – with roots centuries, or more, deep – others are more recent. And it is in these places that nations are imagined: nations start as conversations, born from our imagination of what might come to be. We sit around tables, plotting, scheming, imagining, building coalitions of the like-minded, all to bring the nation into being. In other words, we talk, we listen, we exchange information, we allow the deliberation of the group to update what we believe.

One notable feature of our nations is the existence of numerous formal and informal institutions, such as those for making law. There are many non-state institutions too – churches, sporting associations, political parties. Institutions and institutional theory are usually studied within sociology or political science, where the focus is on their evolution, legitimacy and powers, for example. It is possible to step a little further back and look at institutions through a different lens. Institutions are a peculiarly human knowledge community. I propose that we should think of them explicitly as shared realities where we do cognitive work together. This 'cognitive view' of institutions suggests that interacting persons are necessary to support their continued existence.

I once had the disagreeable, if memorable, experience of walking through a large open-plan office block to a meeting with some colleagues working in a large multinational corporation. A whole division had been made redundant. The computers were still on the desks; there were filing cabinets, bookshelves, documents in folders, for the removal team had yet to arrive to disassemble the divisional detritus. The place was dead, the air was still, the corridors echoed only to our footsteps and conversation. The rules, laws, standardised procedures were no more, as the people were no more. The same would have been true if everyone was present but rendered unconscious because of a general gaseous anaesthetic: interacting human brains and bodies are required to animate an institution.

Institutions have formal and informal decision-making processes, as well as explicit and tacit repositories of memory supporting norms, customs and practices. In turn, these shared cognitive processes (decision making, memories) allow the institution to adapt and survive. When these processes fail, institutions also fail. Particular norms and processes may be declared as part of the formal rule set guiding the institution, but workarounds and tacit knowledge provided by one colleague to another may be required to make the processes within the institution function. 'Working to rule' is when employees stop following certain informal rules and procedures and observe the formal rules strictly, causing delays and inefficiencies in the workplace, usually as a form of protest or a collective bargaining strategy. It is an effective form of collective action on behalf of the workers: this is why the 'work to rule' threat is so potent. Those who manage institutions know that if members of the institution work explicitly according to the rulebook, the day-to-day operation of the institution will grind to a halt. Hence, the recognition of 'custom and practice' as a major factor when the new member learns how the institution functions in practice – as is gossip about the status of individuals populating roles within the institution.

A straightforward (but not obvious) conclusion is this: human cognition has unique communicative, imaginative, prospective and collective functions. And, simply put, these abstract abilities of ours allow us to construct shared cognitive realities. No troop of chimpanzees or pride of lions or swarm of locusts will ever sit in a deliberative chamber (like a parliament or a board meeting) to represent others and hash out *together* a course for the future. Nor will they sit and collectively pass a motion of praise or sanction, and communicate that to another collective entity. Nor will they ever institutionalise such processes, agree to abide by them, bind themselves to them and then act as if they are real and substantial things out there in the world. They are products of thinking, cognitive constructs, but no less real for all that – because of this unique human capacity we all have for creating and acting upon shared cognitive realities.

*

We generally trust what people tell us, and we especially trust those with whom we have a positive social or parasocial relationship, or those whom we identify with in some way. A parasocial relationship is a felt psychological relationship where people come to regard individuals they have never met as friends, indeed as important people in their mental lives, whom they trust. This is not always the case – we also defer to certain types of expertise, especially credentialled expertise. There is a reason why doctors and other professionals display so prominently their degrees and other awards: we laypeople will use these awards as assurance of their expert knowledge. When your dentist assures you that you should use toothpaste and brush your teeth several times a day, because this will prevent tooth decay, you have compelling reasons to take the dentist's assertions seriously. If you do not, the price you may pay may be painful and disfiguring – the loss of your teeth. Moreover, you can test, empirically, the truth of what your dentist asserts. The credentials your dentist provides attest to their long period of training, apprenticeship and capacity to deploy their knowledge safely on your behalf. If they recommend the use of sugared candies to prevent tooth decay, you might find yourself looking askance at them.

And when politicians make assertions about health-related matters? You need to think carefully about their knowledge base: as when former US President Donald Trump asserted that Covid-19 could be treated by injecting disinfectants:[7] 'I see the disinfectant, where it knocks it out in one minute. And is there a way we can do something like that, by injection inside or almost a cleaning . . . ?'* Or when the former President of Brazil declared that Covid-19 is 'just a little flu'.[8] The lethality of Covid and the excess deaths it caused were, of course, greater than is the case with the flu:[9]† You have a choice: do you listen to the voice of those with hard-won empirical knowledge, or do you follow the lead of someone with whom you might socially and politically identify, and on whose continued political success you might financially depend? Choose carefully.

* At least, that's what I think he was trying to say. I have tried to make sense of this remark, but have found it hard to follow.
† Something that never made sense to me about the flu comparison: the flu is in circulation already, and kills a certain fraction of the population annually. It is not a benign disease. Covid, even if it killed at the same rate as the flu, would add to the overall death toll caused by infectious respiratory diseases: even more people would be dead than usual. Why is this okay? It's not. We should be trying to avoid having people die needlessly. Let's not be morally abhorrent about this.

We may, as individuals, have detailed knowledge in a small number of areas, and for everything else we rely on the expertise of others. Jobs as different as plumbing or debugging code on a modern computer system are not the domains of the tinkering amateur. Debugging code requires great expertise, as does correctly pressurising a trap seal in a plumbing system. Bullshitting about your debugging or plumbing expertise but being unable to demonstrate your expertise will make you a laughing stock. Doing so about infectious diseases is likely to be much more dangerous.

Groups play an important role in moderating the memories of individuals who are part of those groups. The group consensus about what has happened powerfully affects the memory an individual has of what actually happened. We are poor at distinguishing our knowledge (that which we know) from knowledge that our community knows. We can succumb to a 'contagious sense of understanding': where a salient but complicated issue is being discussed, we think we understand the complexities better than we do.[10] How many people truly, deeply understand the interactions between the physics and chemistry of atmospheric CO_2 and climate change? How many could write the equations describing these relations? We might know just about enough to have an opinion, but probe a little harder and our knowledge of physics and chemistry runs out pretty quickly. Instead, we seek assurance and knowledge from others who sit at the boundaries of our own knowledge, and these others may not be experts, but may be smooth, polished, high-status individuals whose word we rely upon. There is a clear danger here, isn't there? Especially if you are a politician who thinks it okay to have had enough of 'experts', especially when those experts might lead you to conclusions denying your favoured but empirically unfounded and political or ideological claims.[11]

The cognitive psychologist Nathaniel Rabb and his colleagues argue that what you know – *your knowledge* – is 'collective' in at least two senses.[12] Your knowledge often comes from what other people tell you, their testimonies, which you more or less accept. To use other people's testimonies in order to do something, if even only to repeat what they say, requires us to accept across a great many circumstances that what the other person says is true or accurate (or at least reflects the world as they see it). To put it another way, much of the knowledge we express – the information we have stored in our memories – is collective in the sense that it derives from what other people know. Rabb and his colleagues describe this as a kind of 'epistemic dependence' – we rely on others to tell us what things mean, and what we should value. We rely on what other people tell us, perhaps because they are credentialled, or perhaps because they have widely recognised and demonstrated expertise, or perhaps because they have merely been elected to high political office or have a particular social status (e.g. social media influencers) or whatever. To trust the judgement of the group requires moderating what you think according to what you believe the group thinks. The group's knowledge may not be well founded, of course: in fact, it can even be catastrophically ill founded. In some contexts, this matters not a whit (although it might feel otherwise to you!): your group's judgement about the playing abilities of an opposing basketball team, in the end, is not really a matter of life or death. However, your group's judgement about the likelihood of airborne, respiratory system-targeting viruses spreading in closed, confined, badly ventilated spaces, or about the utility of mask wearing or about the likely efficacy of vaccines, might very well be.[13]

We humans have a peculiar cognitive bias, one that is necessary for memory updating during conversations with others: we are more likely to believe a claim to be true the more frequently we hear it. This is known as the 'illusory truth effect',[14] and there are many examples of things repeated in the popular media which some people then believe are true. Large numbers of people believe that we only use 10% of our brains, or that we are 'left-brained' or 'right-brained' (both nonsensical claims, as brain damage or strokes show). The public at large have absorbed words and phrases regarding memory like 'short-term memory', 'long-term memory', 'learning curve', and many also believe contentions about memory unsupported by evidence or expert opinion.[15] These include the beliefs that amnesia results in the inability to remember one's own identity (83%) and that memory works like a video camera (an especially problematic and incorrect belief), which is accepted by 63%. Some 48% believe that human memory is permanent, and 55% believe that memory can be enhanced by hypnosis. The general public understanding seems to consider memory as a kind of repository into which knowledge is poured, to be retrieved in a pristine state at some later point.

There is no empirical foundation for these beliefs, but they are regularly cited in the media as fact.[16] Moreover, the more frequently people hear the claim, the less likely they are to be able to remember where they heard it in the first place. Not being able to remember the source of a claim and believing this claim to be something that is widely held to be true within one's community can lead to dangerous and life-limiting errors – such as a country's leader dismissing a highly transmissible and dangerous illness as 'just a little flu'.[17]

And where are we most likely to hear specific claims repeated? Within our own social groups. It's not hard to see how this arises: deferring to, and believing, what those of high status may say is a universal feature of human groups. And we may believe what they say, even if it's palpably ridiculous. Moreover, specialisation of labour – whether physical or knowledge-based – requires that we trust in the expertise of others.

We, as individuals, come to rely on the knowledge and expertise of others: the 'knowledge that supports many of our beliefs and attitudes resides not in our heads but in a community of knowledge constituted by other people, artefacts and information repositories (for example, libraries or the internet)'.[18] Many of the beliefs and attitudes that shape our thinking are not solely based on our own personal knowledge, but are shaped and supported by a community of knowledge consisting of other people, tools and information sources such as libraries or the internet: the external environment plays an important role shaping and influencing individual cognitive processes.

We are each, in the most intimate way possible, in each other's heads, for we rely on each other's knowledge and expertise, implicitly and explicitly, all of the time. When we take a plane to somewhere, we rely absolutely on our belief that the pilot, co-pilot and flight crew have the training and expertise for what they are doing. By the same token, if there is a medical incident on the plane and the flight crew call for the presence of someone who is medically trained, they in turn rely on the body of expertise the person who volunteers purports to have.

To put it bluntly, we trust each other all the time in accepting expertise we believe the other person has. As the inventor Thomas Edison was alleged to have said: 'I regard it as a criminal waste of time to go through the slow and painful ordeal of ascertaining things for one's self if these same things have already been ascertained and made available by others.'[19] We trust the conclusions of our groups as a shortcut where we lack knowledge or expertise, and we continually use this knowledge to form judgements about the members of our social worlds. Moreover, we trust in the conclusions of our groups when we don't have enough information ourselves to make a judgement – and we do so because, most of the time, this is a fair enough shortcut.[20] This is, in part, why people are willing to accept 'fake news' in their own social group. Individual knowledge is unstable: being part of a knowledge community allows you to participate in society, for you no longer need to rely utterly on your own frail memory – you have the memory systems of others to draw on too. The judgement of the group then provides you with a cognitive shortcut: you accept what your group accepts; you believe as your group believes; you do what your group does.

*

The social psychologists Jay van Bavel of New York University and Dominic Packer of Lehigh University suggest that group identity offers a 'lens' by which we see the world: 'when you adopt an identity, it is as if you put on a pair of glasses that filters your experience of the world'.[21] Crucially, as van Bavel and Packer point out, groups vary in the norms they embrace. Some groups embrace norms of discrimination, excluding members because of ethnicity, gender or class, for example. But many more groups adopt norms of charity, aid or education. One especially important form of identity in the modern world is 'evidence-based identity', where the group adopts norms of accuracy, and constantly and persistently interrogates reality. Examples of 'evidence-based identity' groups include engineers, investors, lawyers and scientists; you'll be found out quickly if you build something badly, make investment losses, persistently lose in court or fake your data.

A belief in fake news can, of course, be cost-free to the individual, and accepting fake news may bring its own social rewards from within the group – fellowship, status, belonging. A belief that the earth is flat is a relatively benign belief;[22] however, a refusal to believe that viruses exist, when they can kill you, may well be fatal, especially if the leaders of a community, in whom trust is invested, refuse to accept that this is so. Van Bavel and Packer also point out that 'effective leaders manage social identities. They help their groups and organisations develop shared understandings of who they are and what they are striving for, and they unite their people around a sense of common purpose.' Leadership matters – of groups, political parties, institutions, nations. And leaders speak on behalf of the nation to other nations. If the leaders are wrong, the group will find that reality is harsh and unforgiving, and the cost of

belief, of going along to get along, may be bankruptcy, being con-
scripted as a soldier to participate in failed colonial invasions of
other polities, lifelong illness or even death.

*

A consistent theme of this book is that we should think of our memories as providing material for our 'always on' social communication.
We are forever telling each other 'stuff' about ourselves, about our
opinions and about the world, and we are similarly receptive to
hearing similar 'stuff' from other people. Moreover, we rely on that
'stuff' to live our lives easily in a hypersocial and indeed hypercomplex world. We ask those around us if we don't understand and are
unable to figure something out ourselves. Depending on the identity
and status of those individuals, we accept or trust what they say to
us. If it conflicts with what we believe we know about the world, we
are likely to update the information in our memory according to
what our group has told us and behave accordingly, or we might
simply, to reuse a phrase, go along to get along. Going along to get
along means at the very least that we engage in outward behavioural
conformity – we behave as others do. Going along to get along in a
work environment may mean that employees do things that align
with the company culture, even if they personally disagree with
them. An employee may pretend to agree with a decision made by
their manager, even if they believe it to be a bad decision, in order to
avoid conflicts and maintain a cordial relationship. And we do so
irrespective of our own internal states or beliefs, although if these
are aligned (we actually agree with the objectively bad decision),
then our subjective experience of distress will be substantially
reduced or eliminated entirely.

Going along to get along can tweak your memory, subtly, and
without your knowing it. People can and do falsely recall things;
false recall is a pretty common form of misremembering (for
example, a person falsely recalling a car crash, remembering a red

car when it was actually blue). False recall is remarkably easy to induce when there is some form of group pressure present.[23] False recollection can happen because of social pressure and interpersonal influence (this is known as 'memory conformity'). 'Private conformity' is when the person's memory is altered because of exposure to the group, and 'outward conformity' occurs when individuals go along with the judgement of the group but privately maintain their own judgement about what is the 'correct' memory. You agree something happened and you believe it; or you agree something happened and you don't believe it. These differing types of conformity rely on differing processes in the brain, despite the two conditions being *behaviourally identical*. The brain shows specific signals that discriminate between these two different cases, with activation of the hippocampal formation occurring during private conformity – because you have come to believe something to be true, and it is now incorporated in your memory.[24] And yet what you report publicly and believe privately might be two different things.

*

Gossip is one important way we learn about what is important. What we tell each other, what we say to each other, swapping stories and gossip with each other, allied to our trust in what others say, is one of the principal means by which we learn about what is going on in our world. Little surprise therefore that revealing information about ourselves and picking up information from others is something we find, very often, intrinsically rewarding. We exchange information in a whole variety of formal and informal ways. One of the most important is gossip. Gossip is a pervasive phenomenon across all human groups and societies. The cognitive anthropologist Robin Dunbar suggests that gossiping 'is the core of human social relationships, indeed of society itself. Without gossip, there would be no society. In short, gossip is what makes human society as we know it possible.'[25]

We offer our thoughts and memories to others in a social context: one where others are present, in real life, at the end of a telephone, in a video call, in radio show call-ins, in vox pops for television or via social media. As the French sociologist Maurice Halbwachs recognised more than eighty years ago, our social lives often revolve around 'collective remembering' – the stories and memories and legends and myths we tell each other when we're gathered together in groups. One way of creating collective memories is through the sharing of stories about each other: gossip, despite its poor reputation, very often supports social life. We gossip about people we haven't met or are unlikely to meet – think about the intense gossip around the soaps, certain families (the Kardashians, for example) or the hottest new K-pop group. This form of gossip acts as a kind of shared social lubricant, establishing interests we have in common.

Gossiping can be a type of social skill, deployed skilfully to put others at their ease; the sharing of gossip with newcomers can smooth their entry into new workplaces through providing information about norms and standards of behaviour. Studies in hospitals show, for example, that sharing positive gossip reduces stress and anxiety among nurses.[26] A paradoxical benefit of negative gossip is that it can actually police our behaviour – because we want to avoid the social sanctions that come from being gossiped about in a malignant way. Being worried about negative gossip means we care about the thoughts and feelings that others have about us.

Gossip allows us to rapidly share information about others. So important is gossip, the psychologist Frank McAndrew suggests that gossiping is actually a vital *social skill*, because 'good gossipers are influential and popular members of their social groups'.[27] To be a good gossip means you have good rapport with a larger network. The reverse is also true. Those who refuse to share in gossip tend to be excluded from the social group, because they lack information that others have access to, and they are also perceived as being self-righteous or unfriendly. Most gossip in human groups, despite its reputation, is not malicious, and exchanging information among ourselves about others not present is a universal aspect of human behaviour. Gossip is a shortcut, for example, to allow us to learn who within our groups has authority and who does not, who can allocate resources and who does not (or indeed cannot).

Gossip, of course, comes with caveats: it may be inaccurate, and it can be malicious, but even sharing gossip which criticises another person can have very important functions. Defining gossip as 'communicating negatively about an absent third party in an evaluative manner', the psychologist Matthew Feinberg and his colleagues have examined the particular role of 'prosocial gossip', where gossip promotes cooperation in groups.[28] Prosocial gossip can be negative about particular individuals, because it actually protects others from antisocial or exploitative behaviour. Think of this kind of gossip as the quietly whispered word of advice to the newbie in the workplace to 'avoid them – they're not good people'. Feinberg and his colleagues conducted studies where participants played trust-based investment games for points and money. The investor was a confederate who visibly, albeit occasionally, cheated. Some participants were allowed the opportunity to pass on information (via a note) that the investor was a cheat and not to be trusted; being able to pass along this information reduced the unpleasant feeling aroused by cheating.

In other versions of the trust games, it was possible to exclude participants for a round who were non-cooperative (or selfish) players, effectively ostracising them for a while, and this usually brought the non-cooperative players back into line. Even the mere fact of knowing others could pass on information about them was enough to ensure greater levels of cooperation. Seeing someone behaving in an unpleasant way evokes unpleasant feelings, and telling somebody else about the unpleasantness reduces those feelings. Gossip offers a powerful means to regulate how you feel and how others behave.

Does the extent to which we gossip depend on the particular society we live in? One way of thinking about gossip is to recognise that it becomes more necessary as society becomes more complex. In a small group we may all have pretty good information about everybody within the group; for example, within a family, everybody pretty much knows the dispositions of the parents and the children. However, as society becomes more complex, the difficulty of obtaining information about what is going on, what matters, who matters and the like becomes ever greater. So there must be the possibility at least that there are other channels and other means of obtaining information, especially where institutions seem opaque and difficult to understand. After all, what could provide a more wonderful form of gossip than the direct Twitter feed of your nation's leader, disgorging whatever thoughts they have at that particular moment?

The social analysts Loren Demerath and Andrey Korotayev suggest that 'gossip is more important in more urbanised, more stratified, and more institutionalised societies',[29] because there are fewer direct points of connection and information available to individuals. Using a variety of international surveys across 186 societies, they correlated the value members of these societies place on gossip. They find overall that as urbanisation increases, so too does the value placed on gossip. The larger the country size, the greater the urbanisation and institutionalisation of that country, the more importance members of that country place on gossip. They suggest that the 'social order tends to become more complex with increasing community size, and gossip is a means of coping with that condition'. The data they analyse are cross-sectional – the data are gathered across groups, rather than groups being followed over time, meaning that cause and effect are difficult to tease apart. Moreover, their analysis was conducted in the early part of the 2010s, before social media became a ubiquitous means of propagating information within and across groups and societies. These caveats notwithstanding, their conclusion appears reasonable:

because we humans have limited cognitive bandwidth – the limited capacity that we have to process information at any given time – thus rendering us 'cognitive misers', and because we are busy engaging in our everyday lives, gossip provides a quick and easy means of finding information otherwise difficult to obtain. Gossip is a cognitive multiplier, allowing the easy propagation of knowledge through our social circles, enabling us to function more effectively, to judge who is up, who is down, who needs help and who is to be avoided; it allows us to create shared realities. This shared cognitive reality is individual, but can also be regarded as 'collective', as we talk not only about personal experiences, but also about shared collective experiences. We will explore the foundations of, and tensions between, these views in the next chapter.

4.

CONSTRUCTING SHARED COGNITIVE REALITIES TOGETHER: NONSENSE SYLLABLES AND WARRING GHOSTS

Memory has been formally studied within psychology and neuroscience for more than a century now. The case reports provided by Lawson, Korsakoff and others noted, but did not properly quantify, severe problems in memory that their patients suffered. This formal quantification is vital, because without it you can't compare one patient to another, or to someone without memory problems, or track recovery of memory, if any, through time. Nor can you test any particular theory of memory. Into this gap stepped Hermann Ebbinghaus (1850–1909), a somewhat austere German experimental psychologist, who conducted his experiments largely using himself as the sole test participant. Ebbinghaus really got the experimental, empirical study of memory under way, using measurable, replicable and reliable methods: his techniques were repeatable and trustworthy, and could be easily reproduced by others. He described these methods in his book *Memory: A Contribution to Experimental Psychology*, published in 1885.[1] If you attend a memory clinic for assessment – perhaps because of a concussion, or perhaps because of something more sinister, such as a suspicion of incipient dementia – some of the formal tests of memory you will undergo have their direct historical antecedents in his pioneering work.

Ebbinghaus pioneered the investigation of memory by using word lists comprising 'nonsense syllables' – consonant–consonant–consonant (CCC) letter trigrams (such as CYB WSP LXK TPR SSS DRW), or consonant–vowel–consonant (CVC) trigrams (such as RIY SEH XOP QUZ PUY NIQ). Ebbinghaus deliberately devised nonsense syllables to try to ensure they were devoid of extraneous meanings and associations; this way, he could more easily understand the pure foundations of memory. His hope was that nonsense syllables would come without prior baggage caused by prior learning, memory or experience. Ebbinghaus's work has been of supreme importance to the scientific study of memory, while his methodology and phraseology have seeped into popular culture. You probably use the phrase 'learning curve' without realising that Ebbinghaus named and plotted the first 'learning curves' (or, more properly, 'forgetting curves'). Ebbinghaus found that we forget about 70–80% of what we learn within a few days or so of initially learning these word lists. He described other important phenomena: a strong 'primacy' effect, where early syllables in a list are recalled; and a 'recency' effect, where the most recent items on the list were more easily recalled. Think of someone calling out a long shopping list to you – say twenty or thirty items. You will most easily recall the first few items on the list (the primacy effect), and the last few items (the recency effect), and you'll get into trouble for forgetting to buy some of the middle items on the shopping list (unless they're specifically called out and emphasised to you – known as the von Restorff effect; we will discuss this effect again, regarding the recall of the names of US presidents)!

Ebbinghaus chose nonsense syllables for what seemed like good reasons: alternatives such as poetry and prose bring 'into play a multiplicity of influences that change without regularity and are therefore disturbing. Such are associations which dart here and there, different degrees of interest, lines of verse recalled because of their striking beauty, and the like. All this is avoided with our syllables.' Ebbinghaus explicitly drew an analogy with the 'natural sciences' (physics and chemistry) when he wrote, 'we are seeking in our attempt to get a foothold for the application of the method of the natural sciences: namely, phenomena on the size of the effects which are clearly ascertainable, which vary in accordance with the variation of conditions, and which are capable of numerical determination'.

You might very reasonably ask, though, if stripping out all the poetry, associations and beauty our memories are capable of would be missing something. In the quest to establish a truly quantitative science of memory, was something vitally important about memory being left out? Namely, the 'multiplicity of influences . . . [the] associations which dart here and there, different degrees of interest, lines of verse recalled because of their striking beauty, and the like'? Out and out about in the world, we do not usually exchange with each other arcane syllable trigrams, devoid of association and meaning (I exclude telephone numbers and PIN codes).

Instead, we engage in conversation – we tell each other stories, gossip, chunks of information – and we use these narratives to navigate the world. The late French psychologist Paul Fraisse commented as long ago as 1957 that 'We are never alone . . . our most individual memories are closely dependent on the group in which we live'[2] – a view that would have been, I suspect, anathema to Ebbinghaus, but reassuring to others with a more expansive view of memory. Happily, experimental psychology is a broad church, with a multiplicity of approaches available to it – limited only by experimenter ingenuity. One person who attempted to embrace the social complexity of memory was Sir Frederic Bartlett, a genial

British experimental psychologist of diverse research interests, concerned to understand the social transmission and retention, indeed transmutation, of information among people.

Bartlett eventually became director of the famous Cambridge University Medical Research Council Applied Psychology Unit,[3] renowned for its contribution to the war effort (investigating topics such as pilot fatigue and the vigilance of radar operators). Bartlett summarised much of his thinking and his data in his monograph *Remembering* (1932),[4] still an influential book today. Less often recognised or remembered is the subtitle of the book: *A Study in Experimental and Social Psychology*. The contrast with Ebbinghaus is explicit, whose own subtitle conceived of his own book as a 'contribution to experimental psychology'. Bartlett makes explicit the context for memory: memory is also a social phenomenon, supporting our social lives.

Bartlett adopted a naturalistic approach to memory, focusing on the 'poetry and prose' eschewed by Ebbinghaus, using stories unlikely to be familiar to his participant population, namely Cambridge undergraduates. The scenes evoked, the characters presented and the assumptions prevailing were likely to be at variance with the day-to-day experience and cultural background of the undergraduate population that he worked with.

His most famous experiments examined recall of the Native American story 'The War of the Ghosts'. The story itself was handed down within Native American oral traditions, and therefore is a story preserving an important cultural memory, one which would bind together the individuals who listened to that story, and who, in turn, would pass the story onward.

This tale is as follows:

One night two young men from Egulac went down to the river to hunt seals and while they were there it became foggy and calm. Then they heard war-cries, and they thought: 'Maybe this is a war-party.' They escaped to the shore, and hid behind a log. Now canoes came up, and they heard the noise of paddles, and saw one canoe coming up to them. There were five men in the canoe, and they said:

'What do you think? We wish to take you along. We are going up the river to make war on the people.'

One of the young men said, 'I have no arrows.'

'Arrows are in the canoe,' they said.

'I will not go along. I might be killed. My relatives do not know where I have gone. But you', he said, turning to the other, 'may go with them.'

So one of the young men went, but the other returned home.

And the warriors went on up the river to a town on the other side of Kalama. The people came down to the water and they began to fight, and many were killed. But presently the young man heard one of the warriors say, 'Quick, let us go home: that Indian has been hit.' Now he thought: 'Oh, they are ghosts.' He did not feel sick, but they said he had been shot.

So the canoes went back to Egulac and the young man went ashore to his house and made a fire. And he told everybody and said: 'Behold I accompanied the ghosts, and we went to fight. Many of our fellows were killed, and many of those who attacked us were killed. They said I was hit, and I did not feel sick.'

He told it all, and then he became quiet. When the sun rose he fell down. Something black came out of his mouth. His face became contorted. The people jumped up and cried.

He was dead.[5]

Bartlett would ask his participants to read the story, and after variable intervals, asked them to retell the story. He would use these records to try and understand what his participants remembered of this complex and, to the typical pre-war Cambridge undergraduate, somewhat alien and most probably unknown story. Hence the simplification and translation of the components of the stories into idioms that were more familiar to his undergraduates. Simplification and schematisation of the message often happens, as information consistent with what people already know is more likely to be passed on than information that is somewhat unfamiliar.[6]

Now – pause! Answer the following questions on Bartlett's story – and don't turn back to get the answers.

1. What were the young men doing?
2. What number of warriors were there?
3. Was there a boat?
4. Where were the bows and arrows?
5. Why were they going downriver?
6. What was the story about?

Now go back and check your answers.[7]

Did you make mistakes in recalling the detail of the story? If so, you're not alone. Bartlett found his undergraduates made many mistakes. Messages become gradually transmuted into forms that make the subsequent telling of these message to others easier, but transmuted by the listener on the basis of what they already know, or what they think the other person knows. A reference to a less familiar word such as 'canoe' might, in a subsequent retelling, become 'boat'. Did you remember 'canoe' or 'boat'?

Narratives allow the selection of common elements from memory, elements held across individuals and sustained within identity groups. These identity groups might be football clubs, political parties, trade associations, nations. The key point is that narratives work in a way recitation of bare facts (or, indeed, of nonsense syllables) does not, for narratives impose structure, order, meaning and context upon things to be remembered. Narratives animate one's own nation's story in a way a table of dates and events never could. And this telling of 'history as story' makes the work of memory, and of remembering the nation's story together, easier and simpler and schematises it.

The French sociologist Maurice Halbwachs (1877–1945),

whom we met in the last chapter, pioneered the study of 'collective memory', doing so by drawing largely on the humanities rather than the empirical sciences. Halbwachs died in Buchenwald concentration camp in February 1945, aged sixty-eight, just a few months before the liberation of that camp, having been deported there for protesting against the Gestapo's arrest of his Jewish father-in-law.

Working at around the same time as Bartlett, Halbwachs was to make a very distinctive contribution to the study of memory. Using the term 'collective memory' (la mémoire collective), he claimed that 'our recollections depend on those of all our fellows and on the great frameworks of the memory of society'.[8] This claim gives primacy to memory frameworks deriving from society itself, rather than memory frameworks being built upon the individuals within society. Halbwachs wrote that society 'obligates people not just to reproduce in thought previous events of their lives, but also to touch them up, to shorten them, or to complete them so that, however convinced we are that our memories are exact, we give them a prestige that reality did not possess'.[9] Here, the idea that our memories are simplified, schematised, changed, 'touched up' is acknowledged, but with the twist that in recalling our memories we give them a standing or privilege not originally present. We tell and retell our memories in conversation, selecting and amplifying certain components of our memories, de-emphasising others, depending on to whom, where and when we are speaking.

The question at the core of understanding collective memory is introduced by Halbwachs as follows: 'The same event can be said to be capable of touching several different types of collective memory simultaneously. But is it really one and the same event, if each of these ways of thinking conceives of it in its own way and translates it into its own language?' Take a family who went on holiday together. Each family member had their own individual experiences – their own idiosyncratic activities, who they spent time with and what they liked, disliked or found interesting.

However, the family also have shared holiday memories – the place where they holidayed, the food they ate and their experiences as a group. The question then is: can we have memories held in common between us, despite the differences between us in how we might experience, discuss and recall the events we each simultaneously have experienced together? Take our holidaying family – the answer must be 'yes' at some level. Each family member has their own idiosyncratic and singular memories, and they will also have memories that they share with everyone else, memories that are common to all. But these memories, unless written down, told to others or otherwise recorded, are not independent of the memory systems of each of the family members. These are empirical matters, and Halbwachs devoted little attention to them. He, of course, could not know of the advances that would take place in our understanding of human memory, nor did he pay much attention to what had been happening in experimental psychology since the time of Ebbinghaus.

Halbwachs argues that collective memory somehow supplies the schema (the simplified, abstract gist of what has happened), and individual memory is moulded by that schema. He says 'that the mind reconstructs its memories under the pressure of society ... that this causes the mind to transfigure the past'. The problem with this view, of course, is that it attempts to divorce the schema from the brains and bodies of individuals who make up the society from which a culture is derived. The influential sociologist Michael Schudson later restated this view as follows: 'memory is social ... it is located in institutions rather than in individual human minds in the form of rules, laws, standardized procedures, and records, a whole set of cultural practices through which people recognize a debt to the past'.[10] Others argue similarly: collective memory consists of the 'publicly available symbols formed and maintained by society'.[11] But society is composed of individuals and their groups: and these individuals and groups decide what symbols to maintain, to venerate, to ignore and to remove.

There is a (seemingly) profound tension between the idea that memory is 'in the brain' and the idea that memory is 'in the world', somehow independent of humans. I regard this as an absurd distinction: memory emerges from the interaction between the brain and the world. And remember, in the case of amnesia, memory is lost and the person's ability to interact with the world is diminished, to a greater or lesser extent, perhaps irreversibly. Memories are only possible because of activity in differing brain regions, and they depend on the neuroplasticity – the change in brain connections arising from experience – of the differing brain systems that make memory possible.[12] But our memory is also constrained by our interactions with the world – we need experience of the world to have memories of that world. Moreover, our memories allow us to imagine differing futures, to engage in the most fantastical types of mental time travel. The idea that memory exists 'out there in the world' is one that focuses on the past, and is not connected to other processes which memory is central to, such as imagination and social communication. This notion also fails any test of epistemic legibility: we need to be able to understand what is in the world (as Erik Hoel's test of 'epistemic inaccessibility' demonstrates, which we discuss below). Furthermore, our memories actually enable us to adapt to the present and anticipate the future.

In this book I occasionally ask you to try and imagine what it is like to suffer from amnesia – to lose your enduring record of the memories of your life. Moreover, you have to imagine being unable to learn new rules, laws or standardised procedures. This simple exercise demonstrates that there can be no rules, laws, standardised procedures and records without individually exercised cognition and memory. If every member of a particular society (or territory or nation) were to be simultaneously afflicted with amnesia selectively affecting their semantic and autobiographical knowledge, the rules, laws, standardized procedures, records, signs, symbols and artefacts of their own culture would suddenly become uninterpretable and illegible to them.

In a nicely ironic take on this idea, the novelist and neuroscientist Erik Hoel muses on what he calls the 'epistemological inaccessibility' of elements of our past – our inability to understand the rules, signs, symbols of the past, because we lack the knowledge required to engage with them.[13] Hoel writes that 'Art's meaning decays over time just as much as bricks are eroded and entropy does its work on wood. Go see any medieval triptych in a museum, or find any old church frieze. It'll be beautiful and strange. You'll probably have no idea what it means. You, like me, are an uneducated barbarian. At least along the axes the artists were expecting. Medieval art, richly steeped in biblical lore, is *epistemologically inaccessible* to most modern viewers. What was a shared language is now lost' (emphasis added). The meaning of these signs and symbols – created to act as a kind of collective memory for a preliterate people – has, ironically, become inaccessible to a literate people. These signs and symbols have no independent epistemologically accessible existence; they require individual bodies and brains engaged in learning, memory, context and culture for their meaning to survive.

*

I've discussed collective memory without giving it a more modern definition. A useful one is provided by the psychologists Henry (Roddy) Roediger and Magdalena Abel, who define collective memory as 'a form of memory that is shared by a group and of central importance to the social identity of the group's members'.[14] This definition suggests that collective memory can be a body of knowledge, an attribute, a fact or a process. These differing ways of thinking about collective memory allow us to build upon the processes identified by Ebbinghaus, Bartlett and Halbwachs. In regard to collective memory as a body of knowledge, Roediger and Abel see this as a kind of commonly held aggregate body of knowledge about the world, the sort of semantic memory we all hold in common within the particular culture or country we happen to live in.

For an American, this kind of knowledge might be knowing who the current US president is, and at least some, or many, of the names of that president's predecessors (maybe even all the way back to the first president, George Washington). A transnational example of the same kind of knowledge would be the expectation that a Catholic in the United States or a Catholic living in Japan would be expected to know the name of the current pope, of his predecessor and of at least some of the predecessor popes, all the way back to the first pope, St Peter. We might not necessarily have the same expectation of a Japanese devotee of Shinto resident in Japan, whereas a Japanese devotee of Shinto resident in Rome might be expected to be able to name at least the current pope.

In a test of this kind of commonly held knowledge, the psychologists Roddy Roediger and Andrew DeSoto examined recall for the names of US presidents among college students across an approximately thirty-five-year time period, at three separate sampling intervals: first in 1974, then in 1991 and finally in 2009.[15] The students were asked to recall the names of the US presidents in the correct order, starting with the first president, George Washington, all the way up to the then current president. In a rather wonderful vindication of Ebbinghaus's work, the effects Ebbinghaus described for the learning of word lists also pertained to the memory of US presidents' names. There is a strong primacy effect, where the early presidents are remembered very well (Washington, Adams, Jefferson); there is also strong recency effect, where the presidents who are most recently in office are also most easily recalled (Clinton, Bush, Obama – as at 2009). The recall and forgetting curves were very similar to those for nonsense syllables originally described by Ebbinghaus.

Imagine highlighting a single item in the middle of a grocery list: recall for this item will be increased (a 'recall bump') compared with the adjacent items on the list. This recall bump representing better recall for highlighted or salient mid-list items is known as the 'von Restorff effect', named for the German psychiatrist Hedwig von Restorff, who originally described it.[16] In the case of presidents, the von Restorff effect foregrounded a particularly significant or salient president recalled by almost everybody – namely, Abraham Lincoln. These findings are especially important because they suggest that semantic memory, information held in common by individuals, is grounded in the psychological processes undergirding and supporting memory within individuals. Paradigms like this can be used to test claims about collective knowledge existing independently of individually located psychological processes.

*

Human groups universally use story to communicate with each other. We can think of our ability to recall these stories as a kind of 'narrative memory' – memory for stories as opposed to discrete items of information. These stories can vary from fireside chats to soap operas broadcast through the mass media. Some sources estimate, for a US population, that about 20% of our waking moments are spent either watching television or engaged in reading – for stories and entertainment.[17] Our online time is spent reading, watching videos or some combination of the two. Twitter addicts even use the ironic phrase 'doom-scrolling' for the hours whiled away searching for and reading short, 280-character stories and snippets about the disasters currently befalling the world. No doubt other social media are prey to similar phenomena, as we spend hours eyeballing stories, confirming our worst fears that the end is, indeed, nigh. And then we share and reshare these stories with others: we have an inbuilt propensity to share what we know with others – like our medical students after their visit to the morgue – and perhaps especially so if the story concerns something dangerous or is about something bad having happened to someone.

We tell our stories to each other – to teach others, and to learn from others. The anthropologist David Smith and his colleagues at Cambridge University have examined how human cooperation in the Philippines varies according to the quality and type of story-telling occurring within tribal groups.[18] Smith and his colleagues propose that storytelling may have played 'an essential role in the evolution of human cooperation by broadcasting social and cooperative norms to coordinate group behaviour'. Storytelling within groups allows the transmission of collective memories. The stories themselves must be easy to comprehend, easily trans-missible with very high fidelity and transmissible in two different ways: horizontally – that is, between people who are present – and vertically – that is, between generations (because stories are handed down through generations over time).

Importantly, they found that hunter-gatherer stories reliably assist in the coordination of social behaviour, because the stories themselves embody informal social standards we share with each other regarding our behaviour towards each other ('cooperative norms'). Cooperative norms are learned by others through story-telling at social gatherings, thereby providing the necessary bridges from the past to the present and thence to the future, based on the hard-won knowledge of our ancestors.

Storytelling as a specialised social and cognitive practice requires both speaker and listener to possess in common psycho-logical processes to ensure transmission of the story. Generativity, creativity and receptivity are essential aspects of storytelling. Generativity is the ability to come up with a story in the first place; otherwise, there's no story to tell. Creativity involves producing something novel which others value, such as making a story inter-esting and worth listening to. Receptivity refers to the ability of others to listen to and learn from what you are saying, without which telling the story is pointless. Remembering the contents of the story, of course, is vital, or else the story itself would get lost through time. The invention of reading and writing is one means by which stories can be kept relatively pristine and transmissible across the generations. Oral traditions of storytelling, however, long predate the invention of the printing press and the spread of literacy. The development of the printing press and of literacy offers another means to preserve those stories.

In recent years, it has become possible to study the neural bases of storytelling using naturalistic narratives (movies, documentaries and similar material) while imaging the brains of individuals watching these movies, etc. This approach has been pioneered by neuroscientists such as Janice Chen at Johns Hopkins University in the USA.[19] Movies provide narrative and images in a defined temporal sequence unfolding through time: movies are stories. Movie sequences can be easily presented to a person while they lie in a brain scanner.[20] And movies offer specific advantages for examining how the brain interprets and learns narratives. A movie can embody a story, and a story can be told in a variety of ways. Every participant is exposed to the same movie, and, thanks to digitisation, the movie can be broken up into scenes or sequences where the plotline is distorted or randomised, and the voice track is played out of kilter in relation to the individuals speaking in the movie.

Chen and her colleagues have found that during the watching of movies the brain's default-mode network – our big-picture thinking brain network – synchronises across individuals when the 'stimulus is narrative-like': when there is a story present in the movie. To put it differently, the brains of differing individuals respond in the same way to the same movie, but only if the plotline is maintained. If the movie is chopped into pieces and the scenes are presented randomly, if there is no apparent story line present, then this is no longer the case. They can show this by conducting an 'intersubject similarity analysis'. This is a kind of statistical analysis which compares the activity in differing brains exposed to the same narrative and the same movie. In a sense, you shouldn't be surprised by this: most of us are scared in the same way, for example, by the foreboding sense of danger aroused by the predatory intent of the shark in *Jaws*, and the music amplifies our fears even more.

This is now a fast-moving area of investigation. We will focus on a particular study by Asieh Zadbood and colleagues, where participants either watched movies or listened to someone telling the story of the movie she had just watched.[21] They examined the relationship between the activity in the default-mode network of individuals listening to a narration of the movie that a previous participant had viewed and the activity in the previous participant's network. They found the listeners' brains looked very like the brain activity of the speaker as she had watched the movie unfold before retelling it to others. Telling the story of a movie you've just seen produces activity in the brain of the listener similar to the activity seen in the brain of the person while watching the movie. Chen and colleagues commented that recollection 'can elicit brain activity patterns reminiscent of the original event the person is trying to convey, that is, transmission of experience from one person to another'.[22]

Here is the origin of the stickiness of narratives told by one person to another. During the telling of the story the listener's brain synchronises much as the speaker's brain did when she was originally learning or listening to the original story. Moreover, the brain network activated is the default-mode network. This network involves brain regions that are centrally implicated in memory. In a sense, this is unsurprising: memory is at the core of storytelling, for telling stories from one person to another would be impossible were there to be damage to these brain regions, as happens in certain types of amnesia, or would vary from occasion to occasion, as happens in other kinds of amnesia, for example, in Korsakoff's syndrome.

Here we have the rudiments of a theory for understanding collective memory. Collective memory is not independent of the memory systems of the brains of the individuals who are participating in a recollective experience. While certain patterns of activity in the brain may be linked to specific aspects of memory recall, such as being prompted or primed by others, cultural artefacts like movies, stories and narratives also play a significant role in shaping our ability to recall information. These cultural items leave an imprint in our brains and can be easily passed on to others through sharing or retelling. A popular movie may be remembered by many individuals for years to come, and its plot, characters and themes may be easily transmitted to others, through conversation, or even through sharing on social media. What appears to be a 'collective memory' is merely a consequence of the common memory systems of our brains and of the way these memory systems process information about the outside world. And these memories are woven into other aspects of our interior and exterior lives through default-mode, ruminative, mind-wandering activity.

We have all evolved brains and bodies that, to a first approximation, are constructed according to common principles.[23] We now know that damage to differing elements of a tripartite memory system comprising parts of the cortex, the hippocampal formation and the anterior thalamus causes a grave and non-resolving amnesia.[24] The details vary a little depending on the site of the damage, but the overall key point remains: the ultimate repository for information about the signs, symbols and artefacts of a society, and of the explicit and implicit knowledge about how to behave in that society, resides within the brains of the members of that society, but emerges as the result of the interactions between members of that society. These interactions result in conversations and stories about the past, present and future – to which we turn next.

5.

CONVERSATIONS ABOUT POSSIBLE PASTS AND ALTERNATIVE FUTURES

The late Dutch psychologist Willem Wagenaar of Leiden University conducted a famous and extended study of his own autobiographical memory over approximately a six-year period.[1] He defined an autobiographical memory as 'something that happened in my life and that judged on the basis of who, what, where and when is at the time of recording unique and fully distinguishable from all other things that happened before'.[2] He recorded events he experienced during these years – approximately 2,400 over this time – and coded them according to a simple scheme, comprising the elements of *who* he was with, *what* he was doing, *where* he was and *when* it occurred. He rated each of the memories for their salience, emotional intensity and pleasantness. He later attempted to recall, given a cue, all the details of that particular event, or at least as many of them as possible.

Imagine, for example, that Wagenaar had holidayed in Italy with friends and had made a special trip to view Leonardo da Vinci's *Last Supper* in the refectory of the Convent of Santa Maria delle Grazie in Milan. This is an important individual autobiographical moment: *The Last Supper* is one of the world's most recognisable paintings by perhaps the most important creative figure of the Renaissance, and viewings must be booked well ahead of time because of the limited capacity of the refectory and the need to preserve a 500-year-old painting from the miasma of overbearing human visitation. (I was unable to book a viewing the last time we were in Milan – for me, a negative outcome, giving rise to a future-facing, 'to do' prospective memory.) From Wagenaar's perspective, the correct answer to 'who he was with', when presented with the phrase 'what I did, I went to see his *Last Supper*', is two distinguished professors of psychology (Elizabeth Loftus and Jim Reason). The other prompts *where* and *when* should also follow. These are 'bare-bones' autobiographical details, lacking much of the richness we associate with autobiographical recall, but they nonetheless provide the gist of the event.

Wagenaar then attempted to recall the events, given a cue (such as '*The Last Supper*'), over differing intervals from a year to four years after they occurred. He found there was an initial period of forgetting, and that his recall subsequently stabilised at around about 30% or so (not so different to Ebbinghaus's estimates for nonsense syllables). In other words, our autobiographical memories show a standard forgetting curve which stabilises at a particular level of recall (for current purposes, we are ignoring any degradation that might occur from ageing or other extraneous events). The '30%' refers to the percentage of questions correctly answered out of the seven possible for the event (the four Ws – who, what, where and when – and the ratings of salience, emotional intensity and pleasantness). Wagenaar also came to the important and interesting conclusion that 'unpleasant events ... [are] remembered less well than pleasant events'.

Wagenaar's study was of course conducted using himself as the sole experimental participant, so this leaves us with a question about the reliability and generalisability of his overall conclusions.

It is easy to pick holes in a study conducted more than three and a half decades ago which used the best tools then available. Nonetheless, there are important lessons that can be derived from this study. In general terms, his study has held up well. But it is limited in an important respect: his focus was entirely retrospective – he was interested in the *recollective* or rearward-facing aspects of memory.

However, we also spend lots of time imagining and discussing our possible futures. To do so, we use our memories of our past to imagine those possible futures. We talk to each other about prospective mental states – how we think we are going to feel when some imagined event happens; we might imagine, for example, that we will feel wonderful if we win the lottery. This future-oriented imagining gives our mental lives colour, meaning and extension through time. It can create states of longing, motivation, desire: future-oriented thinking and imagining can support the motivational locomotive forces of our inner questing lives. The late French philosopher Simone Weil captured some of this idea in her remark that 'imagination and fiction make up three-quarters of our real life'.[3] While not entirely correct, the idea that imagination and fiction go together, and that we spend much of our mental life playing with ideas and constructing our own personal stories, is a reasonable and plausible one.

Our recall of important events that have happened to us is not so bad – we do, in fact, recall many things about our personal pasts. Cueing recall along certain dimensions (especially the four Ws – what, where, when, who) allows some degree of retrieval of at least certain aspects of those memories. An important caveat must be acknowledged: people's confidence in their own powers of recall is certainly greater than it should realistically be. Wagenaar notes an important application for studies of this type in eyewitness testimony, because overconfidence might lead witnesses to have a stronger belief in their ability to recall events than is warranted. Moreover, he points out, given that we recall the details of unpleasant events less well than those of pleasant events, that recall in a court setting might therefore be the subject of some degree of compromise of memory. Remembering that something unpleasant happened to you is not the same thing as recalling the details of that something – the what, the where, the when and the who. Instead, a remembered sense of dread and danger might swamp recall of the details of the event, perhaps selectively amplifying recall of certain details while blurring recollection of other, more peripheral ones.

If there is one general lesson to be drawn from studies like these, it is this: human memory is at once more stable and more labile than we generally acknowledge. This should give us pause for thought and cause for reflection. Legal cases often revolve around the idea that we can, *reliably and truthfully*, recall details from the past. But evidence from eyewitnesses can be very wrong indeed, as forensic evidence has so often shown. Just because you can easily, under questioning – indeed, influenced by the course of questioning – seemingly interrogate your own memory and give what you believe to be a truthful account of a particular event, does not mean you have recounted what actually happened, because independent, third-party evidence such as DNA or video recordings might show something very different.

*

We assume, in part (and I emphasise in part) correctly, that the function of memory is to look backwards. In other words, we have a kind of time machine in our heads that allows us to engage in mental time travel. We can move backwards on our own mental timeline: we can engage in retrospection. And we also imagine the future: we engage in prospective thinking, where we think about things that we intend to do and must remember to do. These things could be mundane, such as remembering to buy the groceries or to pay bills, or more serious, such as a visit to the doctor to discuss the results of a diagnostic test. We place ourselves on a mental timeline, and we move ourselves mentally backwards and forwards on that timeline. We might move ourselves further along the mental timeline if we are in particular positions of power: seeing ourselves in a line of leaders who have shaped the nation, who believe they have a particular destiny and who all fail to remember that the words of Shelley's 'Ozymandias' apply to us all: 'My name is Ozymandias, King of Kings; / Look on my Works, ye Mighty, and despair! / Nothing beside remains.' What a warning to all would-be authoritarians. We might engage in thinking that is abstracted and idealised about causes we might commit ourselves and others to: we might bring the nation to war. We might come to believe that history will vindicate us in choosing war, or absolve us from barbarities, genocide and war crimes – an appeal to an imagined future, populated by favourable judges, all enabled by mental time travel fuelled by self-righteous and self-exculpatory fantasies.

Sometimes our ability to remember what we have to do on our mental timeline is a little shaky (and that's okay). We use things like diaries, alarm clocks and indeed other people to remember what it is that we intend to do. We have 'imagined future selves', and we spend lots of time thinking about 'what life will be like' if we become something – a social media influencer with millions of followers, a physician who cures people, a politician who determines the future of the nation, a scientist who discovers something fundamental about how the world works. And this is where feedback from our socials groups is fundamental: the group can moderate and correct the fantasies of individual thinking.

We think about what our 'future imagined self' is going to be like, and we will usually imagine the future to be wonderful – we have an 'optimism' bias. Few of us imagine that, in the future, we will be divorced, bankrupt or living on the street. We refuse to consider that our proposed war of colonial conquest might go awry. Our possible future self is a stranger to many of us – and it is a possible future self simply because we have not yet become that future self yet. This is because we are poor at predicting how we will feel in the future; what we can imagine about our future selves is limited:[4] a study of over 19,000 people of various ages, measuring their personalities, values and preferences, asked participants how much they had changed in the past decade and how much they expected to change in the next decade. All age groups believed they had changed a lot in the past, but would change relatively little in the future (this is called the 'end of history illusion'). We find ourselves with a paradox: not only are our 'experiencing selves' and 'remembering selves' strangers to each other,[5] so too are our experiencing selves and our possible 'future selves'.

*

Henry Molaison was severely impaired in looking backwards through memory; it is now known that patients with certain types of dementia have great difficulty in looking forward in time. Work by the cognitive neuroscientist Muireann Irish,[6] conducted both at Trinity College Dublin and at the University of Sydney, for example, has shown that people with Alzheimer's disease not only experience difficulties remembering events from their past, but also have difficulty imagining the future.[7] When asked, for example, to imagine what their holiday next year might be like, or what might happen next week, they offer little by way of detail. An intact and functioning memory is critical to our being able to imagine future events.[8]

The neuropsychologist Bruna Seixas Lima and her colleagues at the University of Toronto have examined how language and memory interact in patients suffering from different types of memory disorders.[9] They focused on autobiographical memory, examining what information patients could recall and the language they used to describe what they could recall. Remember that autobiographical memory requires you to have the brain's memory networks and language networks working in concert.

These two differing brain systems must interact rather like differing parts of an elaborate computing system which allows you to create documents on your laptop.

Seixas Lima and her colleagues focused on contrasting patients who suffer from amnestic mild cognitive impairment (aMCI, a type of impairment of memory for the episodes of everyday life) and patients suffering from semantic variant primary progressive aphasia (svPPA, which is a progressive difficulty in understanding words and language). These different types of patients offer the possibility of teasing apart how the memory networks and language networks of the brain interact. Patients with svPPA have loss of brain tissue in the anterior temporal lobe (the part of the brain directly behind your temples). Patients with aMCI typically do not present with brain-tissue loss (at least in the early stages of the condition), but their memory is generally worse than it should be, compared to age- and demographically matched controls.

There are differing patterns of impairment in these two distinct patient groups. For example, other aspects of cognitive function (such as attention) are normal, but we can predict that patients with the semantic variant of primary progressive aphasia are unable to recall (at least some) information about facts and events. The amnestic mild cognitive impairment group should have few deficits for recalling semantic information, but do show a loss of episodic memory. Studies of this type can tell us about the relationship between language use and memory impairment.

These studies reveal that language and memory seamlessly interact in intact participants, and show how the fluid, dynamic weaving together of language and memory can go awry in particular patient groups. Moreover, when we are looking at memory impairments in patients, we should look not just at impairments in recall, but at the particular speech patterns of the patient – for in addition to memory loss, there may changes in language use.

*

Children carry on conversations aloud with themselves and imagined others, and do so often all the way into their early teen years.[10] The great American novelist Mark Twain is alleged to have said that 'The most interesting information comes from children because they tell all they know and then stop.' Children seem not to have a filter, blurting out every manner of information, embarrassing or not. When adults talk to themselves, they tend to talk to themselves quietly or almost subvocally (and often feel embarrassed if others overhear them). Self-talk persists right throughout life, though: our interior monologue is a persistent feature of our mental lives.

How does autobiographical memory emerge during development? Autobiographical memory depends on two interlocked developmental steps. The first is becoming fluent, and adept, in the use of language, allowing us to start imposing a narrative on our own lives. The second is the gradual loss of childhood amnesia (discussed below) and the development of more adult-like memories. In both cases, the underlying brain machinery matures and develops as a result of experience and underlying developmental genetic programmes.

These genetic programmes control development by directing the formation of different cell types, the establishment of tissue patterns and the overall growth and differentiation of the brain. During early development, specific genes are activated directing the formation of different types of brain cells (such as neurons and glial cells). These cells migrate to particular regions of the brain, and then they transition to being particular types of brain cell in those specific regions of the brain, resulting in the almost incomprehensible complexity of the differing areas of the mature brain. In controlling the growth and differentiation of the brain, the genetic programmes ensure that it reaches its mature state with all the necessary structures and connections. And brain regions mature at different rates: the hippocampal formation matures after the child has learned to speak, resulting in the phenomenon of childhood amnesia. Very often such programmes need extensive environmental input: for example, normal language development requires exposure to a language-using community (family, peers and the like). The normal path of early memory-system development in the brain is less well understood, but certainly requires exposure to a rich culture for optimal development.

Let's think through what we mean by childhood amnesia, its relation to things that might have happened to you as a child, which you verbally recall and describe. Even though you might have few explicitly reportable memories of events that you experienced before the age of, let's say, about three or four, you certainly learned many things: you learned to walk and talk, who your caregivers are, what tastes good, what tastes bad – all those kinds of things. The term 'childhood amnesia' applies not to these kinds of memories but to memories of the stuff of everyday life and everyday conversation. Two psychologists, the late Katherine Nelson of the City University of New York and Robyn Fivush of Emory University, have concluded that autobiographical memory 'emerges gradually across preschool years in the context of developments in language, memory, and self, supplementing the memory systems of early life'.[11] And, of course, this development of autobiographical memory happens in the context of innumerable conversations between the child, their caregivers, their siblings, their friends (real and imaginary) and conversations they listen in to (between carers, for example).

One of the key ideas in this book is that the memories we have and the way we talk about ourselves to others are shaped intensely by the innumerable conversations we have with others. This view predicts, therefore, that there should be a psychological effect observed as a consequence of a person jointly reminiscing and remembering with another so that those joint reminiscences affect the memories of both of them. In other words, jointly recalled narratives regarding some event should enter the autobiographical memory of each individual.

One way of testing this idea is to examine the type and content of conversations parents have with their children, and to look in turn at the effect of these conversations on the type and content of autobiographical recall the children subsequently engage in. We can take this idea a step further: you might naturally expect that different people differ in the type of reminiscing they engage in; in the depth and elaboration of the memories they recall; and in the opportunity that they provide to another person to engage in recall with them. These possibilities have been examined in some detail in the case of mother-and-child relationships. (Regrettably, there has been little by way of investigation of father–child relationships.)

The psychologists Yun Wu and Laura Jobson of Monash University find marked differences in how mothers reminisce about their past experiences with their young children, typically preschoolers.[12] Mothers appear to vary quite substantially in the 'elaborativeness' of their recollection of shared past events when chatting with their children, elaborativeness being the extent to which reminiscences are enriched and elaborated upon.

Elaborativeness may vary from the perfunctory recognition of a trip to Disneyland, for example, to an extended conversation embracing deep details of the sights and sounds, people encountered, favoured rides, food at the hotels, the plane flights and so on. Elaborativeness, of course, can't in itself be the whole story, because talking at and over the child might cause the child to simply tune out and ignore whatever it is that the mother happens to be reminiscing about. The degree of 'positive engagement' is particularly important, as is the degree to which the mother employs open-ended questions drawing in her children, allowing them to make their own contributions to the conversation. Mothers using a 'low elaborative style' use closed questions, with little opportunity for anything other than yes or no answers. Perhaps as a consequence of this low elaborative style, they provide little by way of the rich detailing that might go on in the course of an open-ended, rich, elaborative conversation.

The typical reminiscing style (elaborative or not) and questioning style (closed or open-ended) are consistent across time and across the different children within families. The type, depth and breadth of engagement occurring during mother–child reminiscing shapes, in a very deep way, the child's own memory elaboration. This was true for both western and Chinese families, suggesting that reminiscing and questioning styles are cultural universals, rather than something peculiar to differing family organisations across societies.

Giving the child plenty of positive feedback during conversation is especially important; but repeating and using the phrases and utterances used by the child is just as important to engage the child in the conversation. This method of conversing, which emphasises open-ended questions where elaboration is particularly sought after, has important similarities to the investigative interviewing of suspects, witnesses and others (discussed in Chapter One), as it allows the interviewee time and space in which to elaborate their answers. Wu and Jobson also conclude that the education level of the mothers has a significant effect on memory elaboration, with less educated mothers being less 'elaborative and evaluative' than mothers who are better educated.

Memories of an event are discussed together, and joint recollection necessarily occurs during conversation, ensuring that the details recalled are richer and more detailed. This points to an important paradox about memory: memories reside in the head of a person, and they are tested by one person asking questions of the other person. But we exercise our memory very frequently *together*. A common example occurs when you are playing team sports, where the playing drills and tactics are learned together and executed together. On the playing field, what you do depends on what the other person is doing and how you both jointly remember what you are supposed to do during a particular phase of play.

Another way of thinking about this form of memory is to regard it as 'collaborative' (there is a subtle distinction to be drawn between 'transactive' and 'collaborative' memory: collaborative memory is the collective process of encoding, storing and retrieving information among group members, while transactive memory is the division of responsibilities of remembering information among the group members, where each member is responsible for different types of information – but the point here is the same). Joint recollection of the drills and tactics happens during interactions with your own team and the other team. The overall memory structure emerging is not held in the head of a single individual, but emerges jointly from the interaction of two or more individuals.

Similar brain structures are activated in differing individuals when those individuals are engaging in similar tasks. For example, two individuals engaged in playing music together may experience similar brain activity, and the joint activity itself may feel rewarding, a feeling created by the sense of unity and shared experience. Joint reminiscing – where we reminisce about some past experience together – results in a form of 'dyadic, inter-brain synchronisation', where similar patterns of brain activity are experienced simultaneously by two differing individuals, and the experience of this synchrony might be intrinsically rewarding. Remembering together necessarily emerges from interactions between individuals, and joint recall of memories is a social activity. Conversation plays a crucial role in shaping shared realities, influencing the way we understand and remember events. Through conversation, we can coordinate memories, align recollections and build a shared understanding of events. This shared understanding allows us to co-construct shared realities together, as we will discuss next.

6.
HOW CONVERSATION SHAPES SHARED REALITIES

I'm sure you've had the experience of holding a conversation in which you describe something that has happened to you. Imagine that the conversation concerns a serious incident you've witnessed – perhaps a car crash in which somebody was injured, or worse. Now think about who you were having the conversation with – it might be a group of twelve-year-olds, or a team of forensic investigators, or a close adult friend. You find that you 'fine-tune' or 'hone' your remembering of the incident and, indeed, your conversation according to your audience. The way you speak about the incident depends on who you are talking to, and the memories that you bring to the surface regarding the conversation likewise depend intimately on who you are talking to. You'll avoid the gory details with the twelve-year-olds, perhaps amp them up a little with your adult friend and try to be dispassionate and complete in your conversation with the forensic investigators.

This conversational honing happens all the time, and in all sorts of contexts. You select and shape what you say according to what you think is appropriate for your particular listeners and the reactions you think you might elicit from them. Imagine a different but common scenario: discussing what you might tell your parents about a date night you had with somebody, compared to what you will tell a friend about the same date.[1] Details will be omitted from one conversation but not from the other. A conversation with a close and trusted friend about an intimate date with a romantic partner might depend on other factors as well, such as the amount of alcohol consumed, whether the conversation is private or in a public place where you might be overheard. For your parents, you might restrict yourself to the quality of the meal and the awfulness of the movie, and leave it at that. In other words, the social context matters for conversational remembering and retelling. More deeply, however, our ability to read the social and physical context of our disclosures to others has emerged over many generations of evolution, giving us brains finely attuned to where we are, what we are saying and whom we are saying it to.

Talking about ourselves is what we do – sometimes accurately, sometimes not. We talk about ourselves so consistently and pervasively that we overlook how all this talking about ourselves supports our intense social lives. Locked in our own heads, with unique access only to our own thoughts and feelings, we fail to recognise that disgorging the contents of our memory provides the content and currency underlying social transactions, allowing us to build trust and rapport with others. Crucially, we talk about ourselves to influence others: we want to change or even reinforce what other people think of us, feel about us, will do for us. This is one reason why oratory can be so moving: the best orators elicit within us deep feelings – of yearning, of belonging, of togetherness – through effective and moving evocations and re-envisioning of the past, present and future, inspiring us to a sense of the possibilities of action, of doing something together. This binding together can, of course, serve good or ill: the best orators achieve a sense of authenticity and shared purpose denied more pedestrian speakers.

And how does this binding together happen? It derives from a vitally important aspect of social life – the stories we tell each other, the conversations we have with each other, giving us a common base of knowledge and norms, which draw on, and update, what we know. And much like in the studies of brain activity during the retelling of movie narratives, both speaker and listener are in synchrony during the telling of the story: the same brain structures supporting memory, emotion and language are activated, and even your breathing is affected as you await the punchline. We all guffaw with laughter, or groan with a smirk in response to a particularly bad pun, or shed tears of emotion – together.

*

A common form of synchrony is when we work together to achieve something – and that something can be to try to remember something *together*. We humans commonly engage in transactive memory, where in social organisations and in social dyads (i.e. pairs, such as married couples) there may be specialisations in recall.[2] One person might remember the restaurants from a holiday, and the other the worst tourist-trap attractions.[3] Richer memories result when both parties are actively engaged in recall; and each party relies on the other to act as a sort of external memory device. The social exchanges and discussions result in a shared, cooperative memory search superior to recall conducted alone. Being a member of a couple or a group can have a profound effect on what you remember.

This collaborative (or transactive) component of our memories – where we tend to divide aspects of the task of remembering between ourselves and others – arises especially in close relationships. The overall jointly elicited memory is richer in depth, breadth, flavour and colour, compared to when you have been attempting to remember all of the incident, the event, by yourself. Transactive memory also requires a kind of mind reading for it to be effective. We must each be able to quickly, intuitively, grasp what we think the other person is likely to be able to remember – again, no trivial or small thing. This kind of social mind reading – understanding the thoughts, intentions, desires and memories of another person – makes social life possible. Humans may be uniquely capable of mind reading other humans; it is currently controversial whether or not other species, including non-human primates such as monkeys and the great apes, can mind read.[4]

*

As previously discussed, the group consensus can affect an individual's memory, and people may confuse their own knowledge with that of their larger community. We deploy language and conversation to assist and enrich the recall of memories. Successful remembering together is called 'collaborative facilitation':[5] when a group works together to recall a memory, remembering by the group of particular information will be greater. We gather at our tables to eat and to talk, and during talking we course backwards across our lives, we have a rich conversation about that football match, that wedding, that awful divorce, or whatever it happens to be. This form of collaborative memory recall doesn't happen only around our dinner tables. Meetings are a ubiquitous feature of organisational, institutional and business life, among other settings. Meetings happen in order to set policy; to make decisions; for information exchange. Meetings happen because a difficult problem needs to be dealt with; they are used for problem solving.

At the centre of many criminal justice systems is a trial at which decisions regarding guilt or innocence are made by a jury. Legal systems the world over have in place processes and procedures to assist deliberation by jury members. Occasionally people can't or don't agree on what it is that they think or remember happened during the trial – they have a failure of memory which jury discussion does not resolve. A simple and time-honoured solution for this failure of memory during a group deliberation is for the jury to examine trial transcripts, or indeed other evidence, to aid recall by individuals in the jury room.

Collaborative facilitation does not exhaust the possibilities for how groups might affect recall. Another possibility is 'collaborative inhibition'. Groups can and do choose to ignore vital pieces of information that they could use to make better decisions; they can choose to forget, or disregard, or even suppress, critical information – and make bad decisions as a result. This may happen even though important information might be dispersed among members of the group. There are milder forms of collaborative inhibition, where one person in the conversation simply can't be bothered to contribute much and free-rides on the memories of others.

Silence can be a form of active collaborative inhibition, where an organisation or a group of individuals refuses to acknowledge, indeed actively suppresses, knowledge about certain people, certain events, certain places, certain institutions. Perhaps for reasons of social identity or cohesion, perhaps because of shame, guilt or even criminal sanction, certain topics are simply ignored or not spoken about. There are often open secrets within societies – that members of certain organisations are coercive, abusive, dangerous, criminal in their behaviour, and their existence or their behaviour is not spoken about publicly. Obvious examples are the code of *omertà* within criminal organisations, or silences around secret police such as the former East Germany's Stasi, around the industrial schools in Ireland or around the residential schools in Canada. The code of *omertà* within criminal organisations refers to the code of silence which is supposed to protect the organisation and its members from prosecution. There were powerful silences around secret police organisations such as the Stasi, keeping the East German population at large in a state of subjugation, for no one knew who was informing on whom. Similarly, there were silences maintained around the abuse and neglect of children in industrial schools in Ireland, as well as in the residential schools in Canada. Other countries have their own examples.

Very many societies have, or have had, organisations whose malign behaviour continues because it is not spoken about. This is an especially obvious form of collaborative inhibition, where the dynamics of the group militate against recall – perhaps because the costs of bringing secrets into the light are seemingly very high. Silences can also shape collective identity and thus collective memory – the 'we all knew it was happening but none of us said anything about it' phenomenon. What is remarkable is that these scandals were hidden by a collective silence. Many knew they were happening, but nobody knew how to do anything about them, or could do anything about them. The internet and social media have provided electrifying instances of how these silences can be shattered, and this can be a very uncomfortable process for the society concerned. The #MeToo movement is a particularly important and salient example, which initially blew up on social media and led to the felling, and even jailing, of certain well-known, predatory Hollywood personalities.

Collaborative inhibition of collective memory happens in totalitarian societies. Perhaps one of the most important of George Orwell's many insights in *Nineteen Eighty-Four* concerns the way the Party destroyed and rewrote the past. Without an agreed historical memory, who can know anything? As the Party slogan put it: 'Who controls the past controls the future. Who controls the present controls the past.' The Party ensures that a terrible and malignant form of 'pluralistic ignorance' prevails, where memories and artefacts of the past are lost for ever, the present is shaped by the demands of propaganda *now*, and shared truth and collective reality are whatever the Party requires them to be at any particular time. What you know, what you think, what you can remember is utterly irrelevant – for the worldview of the Party can and will prevail over the memories of any single individual.

*

These considerations lead to attempts to understand how messages spread among members of a group or between differing groups. Conversations between individuals can spread in a contagion-like process to other individuals, with knowledge, gossip and even misinformation spreading like a virus. Conversations can move between individuals, their content becoming widely talked about in society at large. They may even come to be what is sometimes referred to as the 'national conversation'. This widespread conversation relies on shared understandings and shared memories of what is relevant or irrelevant. We've moved here from accurate, if revisable, historical truths to the national conversation – a collective conversation, based on conversational memories, which (perhaps) evolves over time, and where new facts might be admitted, grudgingly and slowly, over time.

What is judged admissible to the national conversation can change for all sorts of reasons. It can be driven by many sources: the media, political parties, even people with a particular status or lineage. Claiming a historical lineage or a connection to some venerated personage or occasion, however tenuous, can legitimate and cement claims by a group within society to power and status within that society. In the case of political parties, it may offer a potential route to power, particularly if a national conversation can be monopolised or steered in a particular direction, not least one focusing on group inclusion and social status.

This is why staying 'on message' is so important to political parties. They need, through the shaping of shared memories, to ensure that they maintain a collective social cohesion and identity, one that is not merely adjudicated by party constitutions or election platforms. Jointly shared memories are at the core of this process. The challenge, of course, in the modern era is that this might be much more difficult than heretofore, thanks to possible message fragmentation across differing social media platforms; there might also be some dissipation of party loyalties in favour of personal followings built through social media.

Note that I make no claim here that *what we believe in our social groups to be true of the world is empirically true of the external world*. There are numerous examples of things believed within social groups that are empirically unmoored from the available evidence. One particularly malign case continues to drive private conversations and public debate after more than a quarter of a century: the 1998 publication in an eminent scientific journal of bogus and unethical data suggesting that vaccination via the triple MMR vaccine was associated with autistic spectrum disorder caused uproar across the world. Parents suffered enormous stress and anxiety, and it took years for the debate to be put to rest in the public mind.[6] And yet, years later, some people persist in this false, empirically unmoored belief – and are putting their children at great risk from measles, mumps and rubella. These are not benign childhood diseases; they come with a significant risk of disability (deafness and brain damage, for example), as well as death.[7] It is known beyond reasonable doubt that autistic spectrum disorders are developmental, genetically inherited conditions,[8] and that there is no link whatsoever between MMR vaccination and autism.[9]

There are countless examples of people believing propositions which are demonstrably untrue. This stickiness of belief has the malign consequence that, as the Russian novelist and philosopher Leo Tolstoy put it in his philosophical treatise *What is Art?*, 'Most men can seldom accept even the simplest and most obvious truth if it be such as would oblige them to admit the falsity of conclusions . . . *which they have proudly taught to others, and which they have woven, thread by thread, into the fabric of their lives*' (emphasis added).[10] But the point I want to draw out here is that this is a belief shared between people: one tells another, and the other trusts that what they are saying is true. And where is the belief when it is not being expressed? It can only be in one place, and that is in the memory system of the brain of the person who holds that belief.

Groups can change the attitudes, beliefs and memories of

individuals who are part of the group. The group consensus about something that has happened powerfully affects the memory an individual has of what actually *did* happen. Without realising it, our memories are moulded by the group consensus – we *conform* to the group consensus. This does not mean that conformity to the judgement of the group *necessarily* moulds the memory of the conforming individual. As discussed previously, there are two possibilities when it comes to the effects of group consensus on memory: 'private conformity' where the individual's memory is altered to align with the group, and 'outward conformity' where the individual publicly aligns with the group but privately maintains their own judgement. The problem here is that outward conformity and private conformity are *behaviourally identical*: you look just the same on the surface when asked if you agree with the group consensus about what happened. It is not possible to determine just from your agreement if you are inwardly, privately conforming as well (and there are no reliable, replicable, usable body-language cues that will give you away).[11]

Imagine, for example, you meet your friends after going to a key football match with them. The discussion evolves over time, and perhaps the group seemingly *now* concurs that a key interception or tackle occurred during the match – which in fact hadn't happened (and which you can verify by rerunning the tape) – and you don't remember this interception. But, over time, you come to believe you do remember it. Your memory shifts and you come to believe something because of the group's consensus – you inwardly and outwardly conform to the group memory. Or you might say you remember, but inwardly say to yourself that you know and remember better than your friends.

However, it should be possible, in principle, to detect brain signatures showing the difference between private and public conformity – assuming differing, covert, private brain networks are involved. One way is to ask if there are unique brain signatures for outward conformity or private conformity that might reflect the stability of memory in the brain. The neuroscientist Micah Edelson and his colleagues from Israel and England conducted a study which allowed them to manipulate memories via social processes, focusing on the contrast between outward conformity and private conformity.[12]

Simulating these processes involves several lab visits – with some subtle but vital misdirection about the intent of the study included during these visits.[13] On the first lab visit (time 1), participants viewed a documentary in groups of five. On the second visit (time 2, three days later), they undertook a memory test to provide the baseline for their memory of the documentary that they had watched. The third lab visit (time 3, four days later) involved brain imaging, while the participants answered the same memory questions as previously. On this occasion, participants in some trials were given false-consensus answers allegedly provided by their companions to questions about the documentary. Finally, at time 4, the participants were brought back to the lab to complete the memory exam again. They were then also told that the answers their companions had allegedly given at time 3 were chosen randomly and did not reflect the actual consensus of the group. What people remember is tracked through time, from time 1 (initial memory exposure) through to time 4 (when the final memory measures were taken).

Overall, participants outwardly conformed to the (false) majority judgement in 68% of trials. When the participants were told that the answers given by the majority were false, they reverted to their own previous correct answer in 60% of the trials. Thus *participants maintained a mistaken or misguided memory because of the social conformity intervention in 40% of the trials.* Despite being told that the answers that the group had given were not correct, participants continued, 40% of the time, recalling the incorrect answers. The group consensus rewrote what individuals recalled. Being exposed to false information, accepting it, rewriting your own memory as a result, comes with the very considerable risk that you will not be able to overwrite the incorrect memory at all.

So much for surface (behavioural) conformity. Was there a difference between what you see in the brain, particularly in the social-intervention trials? In short, yes, there was: a certain brain-activation pattern was associated with private conformity – where there was a now-changed memory after the exposure to the false information in the group meeting. Two changes were apparent: firstly, there was enhanced activation of the amygdala (a structure particularly implicated in paying attention to possible threats in the environment) in these trials; and, secondly, the strength of connectivity between the hippocampal formation and the amygdala was enhanced. When both changes were apparent in the brain, the long-lasting alterations to memory resulting from the group intervention could be detected. These findings suggest that the interaction between the hippocampal formation and amygdala 'may be a mechanism by which social influence produces long-lasting alterations in memory'.[14]

To sum up: your memory system is not a video camera, faithfully recording and re-recording whatever it happens to be pointed at. Imagine a situation where what one video camera records and plays is affected by the mere playing of other video cameras showing a slightly different sequence of events. This is absurd on the face of it, but this is what our memory is like. Our memories are dependent (at least in part) on the groups we are part of. Our memories are expressed during conversation with others, then affected by what we think others think, by what others say, and subtly rewritten as a result – without our even knowing it.

We humans are social beings, living in complex community groups made up of lots of differing individuals, and, crucially, where no one person can know everything. There is no desk across which all social information flows, no all-seeing eye. Nor is there a Skynet – a self-aware, Terminator-style AI seeing and knowing everything and able to predict the future. There is no Borg collective mind into which are all plugged, and which determines our individual thoughts and actions.

Some degree of memory conformity between individuals within groups is probably very useful, indeed adaptive, for the simple reason that social learning – learning from each other – is a very efficient way to learn, compared with individual learning. You don't have to make the mistakes everyone else has made – you can be taught to avoid them. Humans are disposed to trust the judgement of the group, and this trust, in a pathological form, may underpin at least some of the conformity seen in authoritarian societies and groups.[15] Memory conformity emerges in groups, and group-derived memory conformity overwrites memories in individual heads. Others influence our thinking – and our memories – much more deeply than we can know.

*

To be an outcast from the group or tribe, to be boycotted, to be ignored, to be placed in purdah, to be held in solitary confinement: these are all terrible prices to be paid when the group decides to exclude someone. Solitary confinement has such severe effects that the United Nations and others define it as torture when it persists for more than fifteen days. Those deliberately placed in solitary confinement often suffer a profound poverty of content in their speech and in their thoughts. So acute and unpleasant are the effects of such isolation that those undergoing it often hallucinate, or carry on long conversations with imagined others. It is difficult to mimic these conditions in any sort of an ethical way in the lab, but shorter periods of voluntary self-isolation might offer one way to study at least some of the effects of being deprived of the company of others.

The Princeton University psychologists Judith Mildner and Diana Tamir suggest that people are not merely present in the world around you; other people powerfully shape what goes on inside your head, because social context shapes and directs the course of your spontaneous thought.[16] They focused especially on whether humans are naturally social beings or if their social behaviour is a response to the social environment – the presence of other people. Three social contexts (solitude, social presence and social interaction) were assessed to measure the content of spontaneous thoughts during mind wandering. They found, using experience-sampling methods, that spontaneous thought reflects the sociality of the environment, with solitude decreasing spontaneous social thought, social presence having no effect and social interaction increasing it. They also found that people in more social environments have more social thoughts, suggesting that the predominance of social content in spontaneous thought is due to the social content in the environment, rather than to innate social needs. To assess the presence of social intrusions in spontaneous thought during mind wandering they devised three social contexts: solitude (Study 1), social presence (Study 2) and social interaction (Study 3). In the first context (solitude), they brought people to the laboratory and divided them into two groups. Group one sat alone in a room without access to the internet or a smartphone, and with stimuli that did not prime or drive social thinking (things like sudoku puzzles and the like). They sat alone in this room for seven hours, taking toilet breaks as necessary and wearing earplugs throughout to isolate themselves from the sounds and conversation of others. Group two, after an initial assessment, carried on with their ordinary day, having the normal social events and social exposure of everyday life, to be tested later. They found that when kept alone for seven hours, there was a decrease in social thought, but if other people are present there is an increase in their social thought. How did they reach this conclusion, and why is it significant? Previous studies have found that people report that approximately three-quarters of their repeated daily daydreams are about other people;[17] experience-sampling studies find that when randomly sampled during the day about 70% of sampled thoughts are about other people.[18] Our thought has a profoundly social content, so social we are hardly aware of the extent to which we are always thinking about other people, and our status and relations with others. The neuroscientist Michael Gazzaniga says, 'When you get up in the morning, you do not think about triangles and squares ... You think about status. You think about where you are in relation to your peers. You're thinking about your spouse, about your kids, about your boss.'[19] Thinking about others, and about our relationships with others, is what we (mostly) do.

How was mind wandering assessed? The technique is simple: for such an assessment in the laboratory, you are given a boring task to complete. This might be to read, aloud or to yourself, text on a screen which might be less than enthralling. Every so often (let's say every minute or so), you are beeped, and you press a key to indicate whether your mind was wandering during the reading of this text; you answer either 'yes' or 'no', and then you state or indicate briefly what the content of your mind wandering was – was it about another person, or something else? These statements are then analysed for their content. Mildner and Tamir found that much the greater proportion of people's thoughts in the social conditions where they are exposed to other individuals are, in fact, social in nature, but in the solitude condition they are not, or at least not so much. Overall, social thought declined following a period of solitude (Study 1), but the mere social presence of others (Study 2) did not change the volume of social thought. However, social thought increased after social interaction with another person (Study 3). Engaging with others is the thing: the mere presence of others around you is insufficient; being around people, but not interacting with them, does not drive social thinking – in that case, we are 'alone, together'.

A reasonable argument can be made that one of the major functions of the brain's default-mode activity is to allow us to think about others: what we remember them doing, what we think of them, what we hope to do together – all those kinds of things. Our default is to think about our social world and our place within it. In fact, in the United States, figures show that we spend on average up to about ten hours a day with other people – both household and non-household members.[20] These numbers are probably an underestimate. 'Customer-facing service personnel' (to use the unlovely jargon of the moment), for example, perhaps spend 80–90% of their waking time interacting with other people).

We don't notice it, but when talking to others we talk about *ourselves* a lot of the time; talking about ourselves (technically known as 'self-disclosure') comprises a remarkably high fraction of our daily speech. By listening into conversations in cafés and other naturalistic locations, the cognitive anthropologist Robin Dunbar and his colleagues found that about 40% of what we say to other people involves disclosing information about ourselves.[21] In other words, nearly half of what we have to say to other people revolves around our giving information about ourselves to others. We might expect this fraction to be higher in individuals who are narcissistic or egotistical, or those with excessively high self-esteem.[22]

Recent experiments have shown that self-disclosure activates reward circuits in the human brain. The psychologists Diana Tamir and Jason Mitchell at Harvard University have found, in a series of behavioural and brain-imaging studies, that we humans value highly the opportunity to talk to others and to tell others about what we are thinking and feeling.[23] Tamir and Mitchell imaged the brains of people making personal disclosures – as opposed to disclosing known information about public figures – and found that during personal disclosures the brain's reward circuitry is strongly activated. We humans share information with each other all the time. We exchange titbits of gossip, we tell each other how to do things, we advise on the best plumber in the neighbourhood and so on. This information-sharing would be a pointless exercise if we didn't expect the other person to learn from or profit from the information that we share with them socially; as a species we learn from each other all the time.

Sharing information is a pervasive human activity; Elisa Baek and her colleagues at the University of Pennsylvania have sought to understand such information sharing.[24] They tested the idea that we are motivated to share novel information with each other, perhaps for the purposes of social coordination. They used brain imaging to ask what parts of the brain are activated when people had to make a simple set of decisions to read or to share articles from the health section of the *New York Times*. They examined whether or not there were activations specifically in brain regions known to be involved in weighing how much we subjectively value something, processing information about ourselves or thinking about social situations.

During their procedure they had adult participants lie in the brain scanner, where they were given the opportunity to read headlines and short abstracts of eighty articles chosen from the *New York Times* health section. Participants were scanned when deciding how likely it was that they would share the information they had read to their Facebook wall ('broadcast' sharing); how likely it was that they would share it with a specific Facebook friend ('narrowcast' sharing); and how likely it was that they would read the article for themselves. Overall, when deciding to share or not to share there was increased activity in brain regions associated with rewards, with thinking about oneself and with thinking about others. Moreover, there was greater activation depending on how likely it was that the person would share the relevant piece of information.

That these brain regions were active together, to some degree, across all conditions, suggests that, at least under some circumstances, there is a blurring of the independence of one's self from other people – at least from friends – when choosing to engage in information sharing. This, of course, is not a complete surprise. People have long been passing each other newspaper clippings, letters, cards and gossip. The invention of decentralised social media over the past few decades has leveraged off, and amplified, this innate human propensity. Share buttons are, of course, a feature of internet browsers and many people are unable to resist the lure of 'reply all' on circular emails, even though a reply to the originating individual would be more than sufficient. It is hard to know what the 'reply all' is supposed to signal. Does it say 'I'm here, don't forget about me,' or does it signal belonging to the community with whom the original message was shared? Perhaps a mixture of both, with quick replies signalling enthusiasm, and slow replies reflecting indifference, status or perhaps even overwork.

*

Everyday conversations with others are often about the world. When you go to a train station, for example, to buy a train ticket from a vendor, you have a conversation about how much the ticket will cost, where you are going to and perhaps how long the journey will last. In other words, you have a conversation about something in the world that you both experience as a shared reality. We might find ourselves 'developing a joint perspective, or in the words of Patti Smith, feeling [we] share a common mind'.[25] Another way of thinking about this is to say that for much of what we do in the real world we need to enter into conversations with other people where there is a significant degree of agreement about what reality is and how we should deal with that reality.

Imagine, for example, going to our ticket vendor and, instead of engaging you in a conversation about the price of your ticket, she instead attempts to sell you a car, or the half-eaten bar of chocolate she has thrown to one side. Despite your best efforts, you can't bring the ticket vendor back to your journey. Everyday life would become impossible in the absence of these shared realities. In turn, these shared realities require, in two people, the synchronous activation of brain regions supporting social interaction, being able to understand and hold in mind the intentions of the other person, and appropriately retrieved items of information from memory in the service of a monetary transaction.

We overlook how utterly remarkable this kind of cooperative behaviour is, for it comes so naturally to us all. If you look to our nearest primate relatives, you will see this hyper-cooperative feature of their lives might be present in some degree within a nonhuman primate troop. But this cooperative impulse is completely absent between independent troops. You will probably over the course of an average week speak with many people that you will never meet again – and these conversations will mostly be pleasant. The life you live depends on an invisible supply chain of cooperation, extended over many links. Now, imagine a conversation about undertaking a train journey between two individuals suffering from amnesia – a ticket seller and a passenger. The ticket seller can't remember the price of the tickets, how to use the ticket-printing machine or the platform the train departs from. The passenger forgets the destination that they are going to, and even the purpose of the journey. Life becomes completely impossible without the rapid co-creation of shared realities.

We make sense of experience and reality through remembering in conversation with each other. An important part of interacting with others is creating a shared understanding of the world, including thoughts, feelings and beliefs. This is known as a dyadic, generalised, shared reality. Examples might include: two friends discussing their mutual love for a certain band and the memories they have associated with it; a couple agreeing on the best way to raise their children and the values they want to foster in them. The psychological and neural machinery allowing us to engage each other so easily and swiftly requires joint, dyadic remembering in conversation.

The psychologist Maya Rossignac-Milon and her colleagues at Columbia University conducted a series of nine studies focused on how romantically involved couples share reality in everyday life.[26] They used a mix of online surveys, daily diary analyses, naturalistic conversations and lab experiments. They measured self-reports, questionnaire responses, behaviour and the type of language deployed in conversation to assess how conversation can create a sense of shared reality. This allowed them to establish if couples have a shared general sense of reality, the extent to which their shared sense of reality might vary or fluctuate day by day and how this shared sense of reality predicts behavioural choices. They found that a shared sense of reality 'predicted "clicking" between strangers [on first meeting], as well as closeness, rapport, and the desire to interact again'. These factors were more important than the perceptions of the two individuals of how similar the couple were to each other, how responsive their partner was to them or the extent to which the feelings that they have about the other person have merged into their own sense of self (as in feelings such as 'I can't do go for a meal in a restaurant or go to the cinema unless my partner is present').

Thus a shared sense of reality predicts the degree of human connection. People 'clicking together' happens because they see the world in the same way; and this seeing the world in the same way is the key factor in closeness. Does this shared sense of reality give rise to an 'epistemic commitment' – in other words, a loyalty to a shared worldview? Do people, for example, tend to vote for the same political parties for the same reasons because they share a similar point of view? Perhaps this might be why political dynasties arise, because partners and families may foster a common worldview centred around a commitment to seeing the world through the ideology of a particular political party. What drives this shared sense of reality? It appears from the work of Rossignac-Milon and her colleagues that it arises from a shared synchronisation between people during conversation – people rapidly understand that they both see the world in the same way.

*

Politicians of every type and stripe have known that an elegant catchphrase and a set-piece oration can have a marked effect on their own political prospects. The former US President Barack Obama captures the magic of oratorical feeling for speaker and listener when he describes 'a sense of connection that overrides our differences and replaces them with a giant swell of possibility'.[27] Obama intuits that something vital happens during a great set-piece speech: the very best oratory creates a sense of connection, a (temporary) dissolution of the boundaries of the self, along with the experience of the collective synchronisation of emotion and thought among those listening.

One possibility is that gifted leaders are able to reinterpret collective memories of the past in the service of the call of the future; they offer the listener an invigorating trip to the future. We have seen two US presidents, both from the same political party, offer different illustrations of this. Ronald Reagan famously spoke of America as a 'shining city on a hill', and campaigned for the presidency with the slogan 'It's morning again in America.' The promise of his language was that the USA's best future lay before it. A different US president, Donald Trump, spoke in ostensibly restorative terms, declaring that his job was to 'make America great again'. America has been great – and we, the listeners, all remember this (however 'we' was defined) and 'my job is to make that happen for you again' (a very specific 'you').

An old Russian proverb says that 'Russia is a country with a certain future; it is only its past that is unpredictable':[28] the past itself is not settled, but is instead contested. And why is the past contested? Because a reinterpretation of the past is necessary to shape how the (Russian) nation should go forward. Imagining, and reimagining, the future in this way is possible only because the neural substrates of memory and imagination are in a large part the same. This is what gives memory its astonishing potency to allow us to re-envision the future, because re-envisioning draws on the past – what we have already learned, what we already know.

What apparently lies dormant and fragmentary in memory is lying waiting to serve the needs of the present and the future.

Through effective use of cadence, language and imagery, the 'central' speaker – the main speaker who has the most power and status in a conversation or group discussion – can effectively invoke past, present and future, all key parts of a great orator's art and achievement. The key to the power of a good narrative delivered by a brilliant speaker is a story, well told and appropriately paced, which synchronises the listener to the speaker in the most intimate of ways. You hold your breath; you anticipate; you suffer along with the speaker; you empathise; you become mobilised; you are energised and willing to act. One technique deployed by great orators to marvellous and enjoyable effect is humour: laughter is pleasurable, spreads like a contagion through groups (people laugh even if they don't get the joke) and synchronises us together in ways subtle and obvious. Our breathing falls into synch, we gasp, splutter, shed tears, and we do all of this together, for the best experience of humour is a shared one.

This kind of set-piece speech is a common feature of our political and social lives. Across cultures, one central speaker speaks to a group, speaks to a team, speaks perhaps to the nation as a whole. Powerful figures – politicians, journalists and other public voices – can shape the way groups of people remember events. We have seen many examples of these over the past few years, for example, concerning the national, indeed international, emergency arising from the Covid pandemic, leading to widespread societal lockdowns. The central speaker, the person who tells the story, declaims the narrative and alters how people remember the event itself.

The psychologists Jeremy Yamashiro and William Hirst of the New School for Social Research, New York, have examined how the central speaker reshapes the memories of people listening to the speech, and whether conversations among individuals taking place after the speech have some effect on reshaping the initial influence of the central speaker on what it is that people recall.[29]

A central speaker can affect memory by reinforcing already existing memories; or by inducing some degree of forgetting of your existing memories; or by implanting new or misleading memories. These processes can result in 'mnemonic convergence', where memories become aligned and alike in the listeners, because the central speaker can reach all of these differing minds and memories simultaneously, and rewrite and reorder what people remember.

Yamashiro and Hirst conducted a clever study which manipulated memories of events featuring a central speaker. The manipulations allowed them to examine the extent to which shared practice arises in conversation and how shared forgetting may take place. Shared practice occurs when people talk about the contents of the central speaker's message and do so together, giving a degree of practice at recall of the message. Shared forgetting occurs as a result of recalling specific parts of the central speaker's message and disregarding other parts, so that they become more difficult to retrieve, or indeed become completely forgotten later. The extent to which there is interpersonal agreement about the contents of the memory and the extent to which people share common memories can then be tested.

This is a complex investigation, so Yamashiro and Hirst used one of humanity's oldest methods of actively influencing memories in groups – shared storytelling. Groups of participants read either neutral or emotional stories; a single, central speaker then summarised elements of these stories and participants attempted to recall the original stories in either two recall sessions, or to each other, where participant A recalls the story and participant B listens; then B recalls the story, C listens; then C recalls the story, D listens; and then D tells the story back to participant A again. This is an example of the 'serial reproduction' paradigm discussed previously – the story is propagated onwards from one person to another, allowing you to capture elements that are faithfully recalled, as well as elements lost or modified through the chain of propagation of the story.

They found that central speakers can 'reshape group members' memories through selective rehearsal' of particular elements of the stories. Effective chairs of meetings have known this since time immemorial: by summarising the discussion, selectively focusing on certain aspects of it will nudge the group towards a particular decision desired by the chair. Politicians have similarly intuited that selectively amplifying components of a national history can have remarkable effects on how people see themselves in relation to others (most notoriously, Adolf Hitler, in his many speeches, invoked and integrated Norse and Germanic mythology to create an illusory sense of connection to an imagined, and glorious, past). Central speakers influence the reshaping of the propagation of the content of the stories through the listeners. Conversation between listeners also shaped recall, and the overall, settled convergent viewpoint, compared to listening and recalling by oneself.

Hence, of course, the idea that speakers like to gather people together when addressing them. (Perhaps the obverse effect underlies the enervating and dissociated feelings arising from doing lectures and meetings on video links or the like – as many of us have discovered working remotely during the pandemic.) The crucial, shared social commitment to and convergence on the message of the central speaker is missing because the interaction that occurs afterwards – the conversational remembering of the central speaker's message – is entirely missing. One important effect arose from social identification with the central speaker. There were greater effects on memory when the speaker was regarded as being of the same social group as the listeners. In other words, if you regard the speaker as coming from the same social group as yourself, or if you feel a strong parasocial relationship with the speaker, what you remember might be somewhat unpredictable, but what you forget won't be. To put this in context: if you strongly identify as a MAGA/America Firster, you will likely be more influenced by former President Trump than by the actual sitting President. But this effect is not confined to US presidents. It can arise in any human grouping, drawing on the same psychological processes – golf clubs, churches, companies, universities, armies, charities and many more: any of these, under the right circumstances, could become dominated by an authoritarian personality.

Retrieving certain items from memory in conversation in the group leads to the forgetting of other items that potentially could be recalled. If speakers cause people to identify with them in some way, then they can shape what people will recall. A key method for message propagation is identification with the speaker: speakers try to forge a meaningful parasocial relationship with other individuals. These intuitions about the importance of shared social identity are well founded. If a candidate wants you to vote for them, having you identify with them is a very powerful way of directing, through memory, how you will vote. Voting is one of the many means of arriving at a decision by a group. Underlying decision making are deliberative processes – conversations between a few or many people – allowing us to collectively decide on something important to us. How these conversations function is what we will consider next.

7.

WE USE CONVERSATIONS TO CREATE OUR CULTURES

We humans have constructed immense societies, with enormous and restless cities – agglomerations of people, often in the millions or more, rubbing along together, mostly conflict-free, living lives among huge numbers of other people. The construction and longevity of our towns and cities is a magnificent accomplishment, and one that we do not fully appreciate. If we were just a little more asocial, preserving a more or less lifelong solitary existence – like our close primate relatives, the orangutans – our cities could not exist. If we were a bit more aggressive towards each other, given to acts of violence against each other over minor offences regarding our status in the hierarchy – like our other close relatives the chimpanzees (who are about twenty to thirty times more aggressive to each other than humans are to each other)[1] – our cities could not exist. The point is that too much solitude and too much violence militate equally against the kind of easy, continuous, supple cooperation we engage in all the time. We duel with words, not fists; and when we fight, we fight according to rules and

norms. Moreover, we humans spend years developing and matur-
ing, being marinated in the assumptions and predilections of our
societies – our *hypersocial* societies. We must learn the language of
our societies; we must learn the social and cultural demands of our
societies; and we must display this learning day in, day out, year
after year. Societies and cultures are profoundly resilient in the
face of death and turnover of their constituent parts – of us individual humans. We might think ourselves indispensable, but as the
American writer and publisher Elbert Hubbard seemingly said
(although de Gaulle usually gets the attribution), 'The graveyards
are full of people the world could not do without.'[2] We all, individually, will inevitably die, but nations go on and on.

To understand how remarkable an achievement the construction of our vast societies is, let's consider a counterfactual
experiment – one envisaged by the concentration-camp survivor
and witness to the Holocaust Elie Wiesel, when he commented in
an address that 'Without memory, there is no culture. Without
memory, there would be no civilization, no society, no future':[3]
memory is the essence of culture. Imagine some terrible disease
afflicts autobiographical and semantic memory in all the newly born
children in some closed-off society, a disease leaving their sensorimotor functions intact, allowing them to learn to speak (as cases of
developmental amnesia show),[4] to move, to walk, to eat, to grow, but
otherwise leaves them unable to learn and remember the events
and episodes that happen to them during their everyday lives. They
will grow, affiliate with others, mature, perhaps even have children
of their own in due course (there's no reason to assume that the loss
of autobiographical and semantic memory imagined here necessarily nullifies other fundamental biological drives).

How could this amnesia-afflicted generation pass on culture,
learning, collective memories to the next generation? And, in turn,
how would culture, learning, collective memories be propagated
onward to the next generation after that? In short, culture, learning and collective memories wouldn't be passed on – in fact, they

couldn't be passed on. The entire contents of the culture – poetry, songs, stories, religious practices, sports, history, music, politics and all the rest of it – would be lost, for no one would remember them. Without memory, there is no culture – nothing sticks, nothing lasts beyond the moment. There are no enduring cultural practices without interacting brains to encode them, to hold them, to retrieve and reconstruct them. This is not a merely fanciful argument. We lack deep knowledge of the cultural practices, beliefs, stories, foundation legends of peoples where written records are missing. Their cultural practices, their individual and collective memories were lost when those societies were lost. Their cultural practices and their individual and collective memories do not, cannot, live independently of them. Even their very existence might be in doubt, except through the records and tales of others, and the secrets that archaeology might slowly and haltingly yield.[5]

Let's look at this through a 'brain's eye' lens, and conduct the thought experiment we've discussed before, where you imagine you have amnesia. I want you to look out of your window at the streetscape outside. There are signs with lettering, there are symbols on the road, road markings, there are places where people may park their cars or bicycles. There is much implicit and explicit information conveyed by the relationship between the symbols and signs and our collective behaviour. How can you interpret what is going on if you have amnesia? Imagine being Henry Molaison, and new street signs have been introduced, with new lettering and colouring. How would you learn these new signs? Would you be able to interpret them? Use them to build new knowledge about your community? Pass this knowledge on to someone else you might encounter who might have difficulty with them?

Let's extend that experiment: imagine that some terrible disease inducing anterograde and retrograde amnesia afflicts the whole community at once. What would such a community make of the street signs, streetscapes, traffic lights and all the other symbols? Or imagine an invading force who do not speak your language.

The signs and symbols of your society might not be legible to them at all. In the end, all these signs and symbols exist because individuals implicitly and explicitly agree together on their meaning, and they do so as the result of conversation, and because of media presentations, and because of long periods of learning in school and other environments. Signs and symbols do not exist independently of the individuals who interpret them; to interpret them requires a prior body of learning, a body of learning evident as it emerges from the interaction between the individual and other individuals and their environment. Otherwise, to reuse Erik Hoel's phrase, these signs and symbols become 'epistemologically inaccessible' – they simply won't be understood.

*

What is culture? A reasonable definition is that culture involves meanings about facts and events that endure and are shared between people:[6] culture is a set of beliefs, values and customs passed down and shared among a group of people. Music is one form of culture passed down through generations and shared among a community. Religions also involve traditions and rituals shared and passed down among a group of people, Moreover, cultures make demands upon us as shared realities between people, for cultures require 'people to coordinate their daily living with their social understanding about institutions, practices, symbols, and concepts'.[7] Cultures require living, remembering people, surviving and propagating in order for the culture to survive over time. This gives rise to the problem of how stories, beliefs, practices and understandings diffuse through a culture. These stories, beliefs, practices and understandings must be remembered to be told to others, to be propagated onwards (like the stories of the medical students visiting a pathology department for the first time). Stories that show the least violations of people's understanding of the world have the best onward transmission. This is also true of stories eliciting strong emotions. These are easier to tell, and the experience of emotion allows interbrain synchronisation – we each come to feel the same way after hearing a well-told, emotionally laden story.

However, information which is not consistent with what you already know can be very valuable, because it can offer insights unavailable in what you already know. A study including positive and negative results can be more informative than a study including only positive results, as the negative results provide a more complete and nuanced understanding of the subject – especially if the negative results suggest a favoured theory is wrong. Inconsistent information is the most informative because it is not redundant – in other words, it is telling you something that you *do not* already know. This presents a major dilemma. Within a community of believers, finding out what the community believes, and your publicly affirming what the community believes, gives you social standing. What happens within communities where their beliefs are at variance with what is actually true of the world?

An amazing, real-life example of the disjunction between belief and reality was systematically explored by the psychologist Leon Festinger and his colleagues in his important study *When Prophecy Fails* (1956),[8] a book taught on just about every social psychology course (it gave us the phrase 'cognitive dissonance'). Festinger joined a community of believers (self-named variously 'the Seekers' and 'the Brotherhood of the Seven Rays') in Chicago, who were certain that flooding would destroy much of the world on 21 December 1954 – a strong and testable prediction. These claims were based on the prophecies of the community leader (Dorothy Martin, 1900–92), who said she was receiving communications from aliens resident on the planet Clarion (which is unknown to conventional astronomy).

The community, as described by Festinger, was one in which there was a very strong sense of connectedness and social cohesion between all the individuals; indeed, they had sacrificed their conventional lives, leaving their jobs, spouses, homes, to join the community of believers. Their incentives, therefore, for continuing to believe were very strong. Needless to say, the flood didn't happen, and the believers offered a series of rationalisations and explanations for its absence: the 'spreading of light' by the group had apparently been sufficient to forestall the watery cataclysm.

Information transmitters have a dilemma: information consistent with what the community already believes allows people to connect socially. When we back each other's story up, we feel more connected with each other, or, to put it differently, when we reinforce biases in each other – biases we both share – we find this intrinsically rewarding. 'You believe in the tooth fairy! I believe in the tooth fairy, too – how smart we both are!' is a conversation reasonable between four-year-olds, but not between fourteen-year-olds. The step from believing in the tooth fairy as a child to mutually reinforcing crazy beliefs in adults is not so very far, as Festinger discovered when he joined the Seekers in Chicago all those years ago.

Imagine, for a moment, if a valued, important and high-status member of a community turned around and said, 'Actually, this is all nonsense, and what we've been saying to each other is untrue. Let's just give up our belief in the tooth fairy.' Four-year-olds will rebel against this assertion, eight-year-olds probably not. Adults are not, in any way, immune to these self-same processes. Imagine if the Pope were to wake up one morning, declare his atheism to the world and further assert that the past 2,000 years of Christian belief had been misguided and untrue. Will the believers within the institutional Catholic Church or the religious community at large accept the word of the Pope in these circumstances, shrug their shoulders and assume a new posture of atheistic disbelief? Of course not. He would be removed from office and a substitute with more congenial beliefs elected in his place. As the Stoic philosopher Seneca put it: 'Everyone prefers belief to the exercise of judgement.' There are strong incentives in place for a person not to speak like this, not to publicly deny, renounce, abjure, what the community believes. Moreover, even if the person is willing to speak in these terms, will they be believed?

The beat poet Allen Ginsberg claimed that 'Whoever controls the media, the images, controls the culture.'[9] This is not quite correct. There was culture before mass media; there would be culture if mainstream and social media suddenly disappeared – albeit, perhaps, smaller in scale.[10] Culture is learned and propagated through countless small and large interactions and conversations and demonstrations, from caregiver to child, from child to child, from peer to peer; culture is learned from listening to the radio running in the background, from conversations among friends, from the reading of books, from imitation, from teaching within schools and from other sources. We learn, through personal or vicarious exposure, and we pass that learning on, in conversation and in action, to our peers, our children – whoever. And what makes all this learning stick is the smooth operation of our capacity to learn, remember and put those memories into action in the correct context.

Paradoxically, our poor ability to detect lies, misdirections and untruths is the price we pay for membership of our social groups, tribes, cultures and subcultures. Our place in a community of belief depends on our hewing reasonably closely to the doctrines and positions of that community. The tribe offers many things: tacit and explicit assurance of belonging, comfort, security, identity. And when you update your communal memory, you are simultaneously updating your sense of self – where, when and to whom you belong, what you are a part of. And in a modern wealthy democracy, composed of many tribes and cultures, the details may not matter so much. There is a lot of slack, space, in a nation for an individual and their tribe.

*

Commitments to a nation by members of that nation affect what they believe about the relative importance of their nation. If you ask members of, for example, a particular region within a country how much their region has contributed to the overall history of their country, what would you find? Would members of a particular city or region be able to judge, accurately, the importance of that region to the overall history of the country? Imagine surveying residents of London, Manchester, Liverpool, and asking them how much, as a percentage of the UK's history, their city had contributed to the history of the UK. Or similarly asking residents of Mumbai, Bengaluru, Kolkata, the same question regarding the history of India. The answers provided will almost certainly come to more than 100%. Consistently and persistently, members of in-groups overstate the contribution of their in-group to the overall history of their nation compared to other groups within their nation.[11] As we shall see, in the US, for example, residents of a particular state overestimate their state's contribution to the history of the nation relative to other states.

We are subject to biases in our reasoning. These biases arise because of the need often to make decisions quickly and with minimal effort. One common bias is the so-called 'availability heuristic'. This is where people give estimates of something based on how easily that something comes to mind. If, for example, over the last few days you have heard of episodes of crime within your neighbourhood and you are asked if your neighbourhood is a higher-crime area, you are very likely to reply 'yes'. This is because you may base your estimate not on the reported rates of crime within your neighbourhood per 100,000 of the population, categorised according to their severity (as a criminologist would do), but rather on the specific instances that you can call to mind, which you then use to draw a particular conclusion.

If the availability heuristic underlies in-group inflation, then there should be a *parochial* bias in memory. In other words, because you are a member of an in-group, you learn what you know because of your membership of that group and the conversations within your group. Thus parochial bias means you know less out-group information (because you have less out-group contact), and it should increase with the amount of in-group inflation. The more you think your own state is proportionately responsible for the overall history of the nation, the greater will be your bias towards your own state. When people have easy access to memories about their own group, they tend to overestimate the group's importance. To test these propositions, psychologists Jeremy Yamashiro and Henry Roediger recruited 300 participants – 100 each from Massachusetts, Virginia and California.[12] Participants had to be affiliated with their home state (they had to have lived there until the age of eighteen, they must be living there now and they must have spent no more than four years outside the state). A variety of other demographic information was also collected: importantly, participants were asked to rate on a five-point scale how important their home state was as part of their personal identity. Participants generally chose numbers corresponding to the phrases 'a moderate amount' and 'a lot'. They were then given two tasks: on a scale of 1–100, to estimate what percentage of US history was accounted for by their own state, and secondly, to list important historical events that occurred for each of the three states – their own home state and the two other US states. They found that participants attributed 11% more US history to their home state compared to the other states. Participants also recalled more in-state events than out-of-state events, and the more they identified with their home state the greater was the bias found in assessing the historical influence of their home state.

When people are reminded of other groups' memories, this tendency to overestimate their own state's importance is reduced. This overestimation happens because it's easy to remember one's own group's memories, rather than because the group is more important or special. The study gives us a better understanding of why people overestimate their group's importance and suggests ways to reduce this bias. These effects on excess identification with one's own region are a little like the hazy glow attending the residents of Lake Wobegon, the imaginary locale created by the American novelist Garrison Keillor: 'where all the women are strong, all the men are good-looking, and all the children are above average'.

Happily, such biases in recall can be overcome. When you are forced to recall only out-of-state information (ignoring your home state), the in-group inflation effect is reduced. Imagine you are from Texas but are asked to recall facts about California (ignoring what you know about Texas). This forced recall of information about California reduces the effect of in-group inflation, as you are focused on information not about your home state (Texas), but rather about another state (California). Some of the basis for conflict between groups regarding who gets to decide what is important about memory might derive from these sincerely held and almost irreconcilable differences of opinion between competing groups regarding their respective importance to their nation's history. However, undertaking an exercise in recalling information about the out-group reduces your in-group biases, and you might discover along the way that the members of the out-group are not so bad, really, that you have a few things in common with them and that maybe you can get along with them. (Of course, I am not talking here about professional disputes regarding historical events between expert historians; rather, I am referring to disputes between groups, each with their own unique vantage point and their own collective memory.)

Our use of memory here is intimately coupled with the stories that we tell ourselves about ourselves and about our greater social world, including those with whom we identify. And how do we know those with whom we identify? Well, in a very large part because of the language that they use – in other words, how they talk to us, the things they say to us and what we remember about them. Strong identification with the in-group, combined with in-group inflation, leads people to assign greater importance to their own group than would happen were a space alien to cast a cold and inquisitorial eye over their importance or contribution. Ideally, these differences of opinion and identification do not become hotly disputed, and are diffused through rivalrous songs at the sporting ground or through being bound together as members of the nation – another important form of group membership. Who cares about the rivalry between Philadelphia and Pittsburgh? After all, we're all Pennsylvanians, and our true rivalry is with Ohio! And who cares about our rivalry with Ohio? After all, we're Americans and our true rivalry is with—[fill in the gap]! The point here is that rivalry and competition between identities is nested within a larger group of other identities that can be adopted or discarded as needed. And these can be friendships too rather than rivalries.

*

A commonly used phrase is 'culture war' (or 'wars'), indicating a conflict between social groups over the supremacy of one group's values, beliefs and practices over those of another.[13] The British historian Dominic Sandbrook says, 'there are moments in history when disputes about history, identity, symbols, images and so on loom very large. Think about so much of 17th-century politics, for example, when people would die over the wording of a prayer book.'[14] A culture war is a peculiar form of conflict, appealing principally to the emotions: it is a conflict where one group is terribly upset about *what its members think other people think*, and then protests over that perception. Whether that perception is empirically secure is another matter entirely, and another debate – but not for here. Culture wars can be consequential, for they represent an attempt by interest groups, some powerful, some not, to engage in a struggle over the nature and meaning of history. The aspects of our history we choose to remember and venerate, and the aspects of our history we skate past – where we engage in a 'collective inhibition of recall' (a 'collective amnesia') – are open and evolving questions. The culture wars in some senses therefore are an attempt to define the terms on which we engage with and meet the past.

Imagine, for example, an alien coming to earth and inspecting our statues – those lumps of carved stone or cast metal before which we humans gather reverentially or antagonistically, or which we perhaps sometimes just ignore. A statue by itself, to someone without knowledge of who or what it represents, is just a carved lump of stone or cast metal; remember the traveller encountering fallen Ozymandias – a statue might induce perhaps a feeling of familiarity, maybe awe at its size or the quality of the craftsmanship, but perhaps not much more. It is what we individually and collectively remember about what those statues tell us that is important.

Or consider a community of people suffering from retrograde amnesia attending a commemoration. Perhaps they might be able to mouth the words of the national anthem, but the profundity, depth and communal significance of the occasion will elude them. Cultural artefacts act as prompts for our collective memory: the presence of a particular statue or the act of commemoration affects what people know about the nation. The memories people bring to bear on an artefact or a commemoration bear directly upon how they behave towards the artefact or the commemoration itself. This is why conflict over what statues represent is so important – it is a conflict ultimately about the values that stand behind the statues.

Note that the act of felling a statue will become part of the historical record. The events in the city of Bristol, in the United Kingdom, of 2020, for example, where the statue of the slave trader Edward Colston (1636–1721) was removed by a crowd and dumped in Bristol Harbour, can be seen precisely in this light. From the vantage point of a century or so hence, the fact that a crowd moved with a common purpose to remove a statue from the public square of a known slave trader will (likely) be seen as an act that will require exploration and explanation. Felling or defending a statue is as much a part of the story that we wish to tell the future about what we believe and value in the present as it is about using a statue or a symbol to present some aspect of the past. Similar debates and acts are underway in many places.

As the political scientist Simukai Chigudu of the University of Oxford puts it: 'arguments over statues are always about the present and not the past. They are about which aspects of our cultural heritage we choose to honour in public space and why. They are about what values we wish to promote and who has a voice in these matters.'[15] I recall once chatting with two English friends living in Ireland who were (initially) surprised that Oliver Cromwell was not regarded as a great figure (because of the Cromwellian campaign of conquest in Ireland). Ireland lacks public statues venerating Cromwell; to this day, proposals (which do not exist, I hasten to add) to venerate him publicly with a statue would be met with derision and incomprehension. Irish collective memories of Cromwell invariably circle back to the 'Cromwellian' injunction to the native Irish that they must go 'to hell or to Connacht'.[16] Yet there are many statues to Cromwell in the UK. Perspective and belonging matter where remembering and commemoration are concerned.

At the centre of these kinds of conflicts is, of course, the question who gets to 'decide' on our history. In one sense, this is a meaningless question, for history is not written, unchanging, for all time. We do not freely get to decide what enters into the historical record. Who gets to decide on our history depends on the context you are talking about. In this sense, our history and how we choose to see it is often more about what we talk about in the here and now than it is about any canonical consensus on the events that occurred and the reasons behind them. Similarly, debates within the mass media about the nature of history can revolve around how particular narratives can feed into certain views regarding patriotism and belonging. It is hard to escape the view that powerful actors with a particular, invested viewpoint resent others – professional historians, for example – engaging in attempts to redefine what the history of their nation is.

Intellectual enquiry demands a lens through which to interrogate history. Who gets to decide on the particular lens may depend on the political and educational culture of the particular country involved. One lens is to tell the history as the story of 'great men' and their doings (though what about the women? Or geography?). A pro-colonial lens might function as a kind of comfort blanket, retrospectively justifying the violent incursion by one nation into another, supposedly bringing civilisation or whatever; the pro-colonial telling will find outlets among the colonisers, but probably not among the colonised. A Marxist lens might focus on the interactions between power, capital, ownership of the means of production and class relations; an anti-colonialist lens might focus on the struggles of subjugated nations to be free of their colonial oppressors; a human-rights lens might focus on the changes in the treatment and inherent value placed on individuals and groups of individuals through the years. No matter what lens it will be, it will not be a 'tell it like it is', for the act of telling requires a prior act of focus and selection.

By evoking widely shared past memories and by telling stories about possible futures over timescales that people can readily imagine, politicians can potentially leverage beneficial outcomes for themselves. Of the former UK Prime Minister Boris Johnson, the journalist Tom McTague wrote: 'To him, the point of politics – and life – is not to squabble over facts; it's to offer people a story they can believe in.'[17] Offering no more than a story works only for as long as divergences between the story and reality do not matter too much. Facts matter – as every politician finds out in the end.

Refracting memory through the lens of rose-tinted retrospection might elicit especially strong responses from some older voters, who are already inclined to biased recall of the past, and might even be mobilised effectively by feelings of loss. The Czech author Milan Kundera tellingly writes in his novel *Ignorance* that 'The Greek word for "return" is nostos. Algos means "suffering". So nostalgia is the suffering caused by an unappeased yearning to return.' In a different take, the economic historian Joel Mokyr said, 'The Good Old Days may have been old, but they were never good.'[18] Certainly, as we age it appears that nostalgia is an ever greater component of our thinking. Nostalgia is a complex and mixed emotion coloured by the specific nature of the memories recalled. Experience sampling and diary studies find that older adults are three times more likely, compared to middle-aged adults, to report nostalgia, and these feelings of nostalgia are both positively and negatively inflected.[19] Indulging in certain types of selective nostalgia can be a form of 'weaponised' mental time travel by politicians[20] (for example, Trump's MAGA, or the Brexiter's 'Take Back Control'). And nostalgia can be incorporated into individual identity via memory. Many countries have gruesome pasts, often over extended periods, and few would want to return to those times (although there may be revanchist voices wishing to take their society back to a prior time, perhaps when their ancestors exercised power and control). The key point is that nostalgia-inflected rhetoric can be used to mobilise, reinterpret and rewrite memories. In effect, those memories are turned to use in the present – nudging voting preferences for a particular candidate, for example – engaging in mental time travel that invokes a future that is effectively an attempt to return to an apparent lost idyll of the past.

Is it possible to connect the psychology of mental time travel and collective memory? Mental time travel is a central experience of memory in individuals. Its relationship to the way a people remember their nation's past might be affected by how people imagine their nation's future.[21] While individuals might imagine that future in very specific terms, just as they imagine their own future lives, as individuals they believe they have relatively little agency in the overall life of their nations, given that what one person can do to change the future trajectory of their country is limited. What we know determines what we imagine; and what we know and what we can imagine depend, in turn, on the integrity of particular brain systems, and how they interact with other brain regions and, indeed, with other brains possessing other memories and identities. If we know history in very specific terms, then we are likely to imagine the future in specific terms, whereas those with a sort of generalised knowledge of the past will imagine the future in more general ways. In other words, individual autobiographical memory shapes individual identity, and collective memory shapes collective identity.

Communities everywhere go to great trouble and expense to construct monuments to people of particular significance, to name roads and streets and parks after important or significant individuals; communities engage extensively in commemoration; and through mass media disseminate information around culturally significant events, places and people. In turn, this kind of information provisioning enters the memory of individuals and is discussed in a whole variety of ways within families, within groups of friends, online or whatever. Thus 'individual memory might be best viewed as a social organ designed, in part, to promote the formation of collective memories'.[22] This is key for the future development of our societies, especially where absorbing and integrating new members into those societies is concerned. A key task for immigrants to a new society is learning the explicit and implicit norms and mores, treasured pieces of history, points, places and persons of reverence and renown, and all the other information the members of the community they have migrated into already know and take for granted. The host community will often have a long process of actively educating, in schools and other places, the members of its own society. The consequence is that 'natives' understand and grasp and express the mores, norms and practices of the society they are part of, for they have been learning these since early in life. They have acquired a huge body of tacit and explicit knowledge they can quickly deploy in social and other situations.

By contrast, the immigrant – despite the globalising of our world over the past few decades – must still learn the nuances and lineaments of the society they are now living in. They need to quickly learn what can be said, what they can do, what they cannot say and what they should not do. The supposed lack of integration of immigrants in their new society has become a touchstone issue for many in some host societies. The mirror of this is the loss the society from which they have departed might experience. In both cases, memory can be seen to be at the heart of the dispute. The departing society might lament the 'brain drain', the investment their origin society has made in educating the now emigrant, and elements of the host society may come to believe that the presence of immigrants somehow destabilises their society, while ignoring the benefits that immigrants may bring to it.

There are lots of ways of thinking about the integration of new members of a society. Economists, for example, generally conclude that immigrants give a great economic and social boost to their new society,[23] bringing knowledge and a diversity of viewpoints, networks and contacts otherwise inaccessible to that society.[24] However, the point here is not to adjudicate on claims regarding immigration. Rather, it is to understand how it is that we construct societies in the first place. Remember, we humans migrated out of Africa, in multiple waves, 120,000–50,000 years ago, radiating right across the land mass of Eurasia and eventually into Australasia and the Americas. In those prehistoric times, nations did not exist, borders between nations did not exist, and passports for travel most certainly did not exist. The world at that time was truly free, in the sense that anyone could move anywhere they pleased. However, nations have come into being through historical accident, through colonial lines drawn on a map, through the raw exercise of power and other means. But how can the nation itself come to exist through time? I am going to suggest that, contrary to lots of theorising in many disciplines, all our nations began as conversations. This is the topic we will turn to next.

8.
OUR NATIONS BEGAN AS CONVERSATIONS: COUNTRIES ARE COGNITIVE CONSTRUCTS

We humans bring imagined, participative entities of great temporal and geographic scales into being – the *nations* of the world that presently exist, the abstractions we are willing to live and die for.[1] Imagined, for there is nothing given by way of commandments from on high to delineate the nations of the world: the present nations of the world were not foreordained. Nations have arisen, fallen, persisted, mutated, adapted, for chance reasons: geography, power, colonisation among them. As you read this, all over the world there are both peaceful and violent groups and organisations pondering the question of how to bring the nations they imagine, long for and offer fealty to into nationhood, and have these imagined entities recognised as *nations* by other *nations*.

We experience this reality of differing nations in all sorts of different ways. Travelling from Dublin Airport to the United States offers a clear example, because Dublin Airport has a formal US Customs and Border Protection (CBP) pre-clearance crossing zone for travel to the US. This is both legally and actually a US border, with American CBP officers – some thousands of kilometres from the more usual international air border in the US. Their presence on another island, in another legal jurisdiction, where this very handy fiction-of-a-sort is maintained means *borders are cognitive constructions* (or shared realities) – they are just inventions of human thinking and action, rather than something given in the inherent construction of the world itself. We think of borders as real, and they certainly are real as barriers, but they are barriers we humans build and bind ourselves to, marking the space between peoples and nations. Moving the border to Dublin means you have no border formalities on arrival in the US. The process is straightforward: you check into your flight, and then you proceed through US Immigration – *in Dublin Airport* – for questioning regarding the purpose of your travel to the US. For some reason, this process always causes me no end of anxiety. I'm standing in line, having filled in the various online forms, and my heart is pounding (why?); finally, I'm called by the American CBP officer, who asks me the purpose of my travel to the US. We chat about the conference I'm attending; my heart pounds a little less, and he stamps my passport and wishes me a pleasant onward journey. And I then arrive in Philadelphia, on the other side of the US immigration border, as if I had been a native US traveller – unlike travellers from other locales. We humans can institute processes that allow us to treat others 'as if' they were the same as us: we merely need to think, agree and act, and it becomes so!

When we cross borders, we often meet immigration officers who have a specific job – to question us about the purpose of our visit, and then decide if we're 'fit persons' to be admitted to their country. And the place they start is by examining your passport. Do you have a passport – or do you have a *passeport* (French); *një pasaportë* (Albanian); *putovnicu* (Croatian); *diavatírio* (Greek); *pas* (Irish); *passaporto* (Italian); *baasaboor* (Somali); *hộ chiếu* (Vietnamese); *iwe irinna kan* (Yoruba)? You get the idea – every country issues these documents according to an internationally negotiated and agreed standard, with your biometric details encoded, an accompanying photo and much else besides. And you typically must have a passport to cross an international border – unless this requirement has been negotiated away by all parties on all sides of the border or borders.[2] And authoritarians love restricting travel, even requiring internal travel documents to move around one's own nation. Passports also have a certain status or power as national documents, as they confer a relative degree of freedom of movement – or otherwise – on the passport holder. Moreover, every year, various rating agencies judge the 'power' ranking of a passport – basically a status ranking, but of a legal document issued by the various nations of the world. The Henley Passport Index ranks the German passport as the number one, 'most powerful' passport of 2021, and the United Arab Emirates at number 16, whereas the passportindex.org rates the passport of the United Arab Emirates as the most powerful, and Germany as a joint number 3. How do these differences in rankings arise? Simple: you give certain (arbitrary) numerical weightings to the differing factors associated with a passport, add them up and then you list them in rank order. Change the weightings and you change the relative rankings; hence there is an element of a parlour game about these systems.

Is there a proper, principled reason to favour one ranking system over another? Not really, for just like passports themselves these comparison games are fundamentally cognitive constructs, serving status games. Passport comparisons are compiled in the hope of eliciting feelings of pride by the possessors of the 'top ten' passports and arousing envy in those possessing the 'less powerful' passports lower down the list. These rankings attempt to engage emotions invoked during social-comparison and status games, especially those of 'envy and scorn'[3] – envy experienced by the lower-ranked passport holder for the higher-ranked, and perhaps scorn evinced by the higher-ranked for the lower-ranked. Passports can be proxies for the status of nations, and for our membership of nations. And, of course, there are the inevitable rankings of nations. (There are at least ninety-five ranking systems, and there are about 200 countries, so I guess there is a ranking for every other nation's preference.)[4] These status rankings seem a bit barmy, *outré* even, when you step back from them and look at them with a cold eye: passports are legal documents, and their issuance is beyond the direct control of the person to whom they are issued. They are subject to rules the individual has little say in constructing. Feeling pride in your passport is, at first glance, a little odd, but, in the end, it is not the document that matters.[5] It is what the document supposedly represents regarding the networks of status relations that your passport affords you. Some passport holders must wait and queue, and other passport holders pass freely; some are privileged, others not. And these things are all subject to agreement.

We can think of these 'nation ranking' and 'passport ranking' systems as a form of 'meta-collective status comparison' – a way of thinking about collective comparisons that asks the question 'What do we (our group) collectively think about *other* groups?' Sitting at home, in your country, what do you think people of the country next door think and remember collectively about themselves and about your country? Reflections on meta-collective memory offer an important exercise in understanding others, especially in situations where there are attempts to align interests in negotiations. As we shall see, when we turn to work by Jeremy Yamashiro and Henry Roediger, the exercise of having to remember the past of other places reduces the bias you might have toward preferentially remembering, and perhaps even privileging, your own place. To put it another way, meta-collective thinking about nations encourages us to ask ourselves: 'What do *we* take for granted about what others think about themselves and about us?' To concretise it: 'What do we think that the Germans (or whoever) usually think about us?' Your job here is to imagine what it is that another nation thinks of you (or indeed how they may stereotype you).

Even the Bible says, 'Cursed is anyone who moves their neighbor's boundary stone.'[6] A mere crossing of an imaginary line on a map – a border – can change substantially and dramatically how a nation views its own past, even for events that are still within historical memory. For example, when did the Second World War start, and when did it end? For France and Britain, the Second World War started in September 1939. For Russia, because of the Molotov–Ribbentrop Pact, what the Russians call the 'Great Patriotic War' dates from the German invasion of 1941. In the US telling, the start of the war dates from the bombing of Pearl Harbor on 7 December 1941. In the Chinese telling, it starts with the invasion of China by Japan in 1937. The end of the war is marked in a variety of ways. There is VE Day, or Victory in Europe, dated 8 May 1945, whereas VJ Day, Victory in Japan – the capitulation of Japan in August 1945, after the Hiroshima and Nagasaki bombings – is 2 September 1945. Other countries again see the Second World War in different terms.

Moreover, combatant countries reliably claim greater responsibility for victory and the war effort than they allow their country's allies: 'We won the war – and no one else did much.'[7] This is the kind of 'in-group inflation' of importance that we have previously seen is apparent in residents of differing US states. The point here of course is that, to a war historian, adjudicating on the collective memories of particular countries is not really the issue. The elements abstracted from these kinds of memorial presentations are what stick in individuals' memories and thereby shape the collective memory of the nation. The collective memory, by definition, is not the historical account of what happened, it is the account of what people 'remember' happened. Recall that collective memories are memories shared, or held in common, by the members of a group, and which are of particular and central importance to the identity and agency of that group[8] (the group can be members of a nation, of course).

*

This book argues that the communal and collective uses of memory allow us to construct shared realities at differing scales. These scales range from couples, families and small groups, supported by and mediated through social and cultural practices, to the larger scales of institutions, to nations themselves – the entities that we will live and die for. And we can go further – to supranational entities, of which there are thousands, small, medium and large, famous, infamous and obscure, venerated, trusted, hated and mistrusted. Mostly, the supranational category does not attract much by way of ire. Few people wake up in the morning worried about their nation's membership of the Universal Postal Union (established by the Treaty of Bern of 1874), for example. It can be the case, of course, that some people do wake up in the morning affecting to be worried about their country's continuing membership of certain international treaty organisations (such as the European Union), or by their country's non-membership of other international treaty organisations (such as the Comprehensive and Progressive Trans-Pacific Partnership, the CPTPP), or their country's non-membership of non-existent organisations (such as CANZUK, or Canada, Australia, New Zealand, United Kingdom).[9] The larger point is that individual identities acting in concert can become bound up in these kinds of cognitive projects, in ways that shape the fate of nations, for better or worse (and outcomes can be worse, but admitting this to oneself and others is hard).

How does a nation arise as a shared cognitive project? I claim that all nations initially began as conversations – conversations where people dreamed of what might be, what resources could be theirs, what could be taken, what could be defended against others.

All nations began as conversation with the like-minded first, the convincing of others, and conflict with others again; territory is demarcated, boundaries regulated, treaties signed in conference rooms governing mutual recognition of each nation by the other. Nations are not preordained. They require imagination to envision. After all, there was a time when nations did not exist, and such borders as there were largely physical in nature: watercourses, oceans, mountain ranges and the like. And yet, today, in the modern world there are about 200 nations recognised by a collective, supranational entity – the United Nations – itself a shared cognitive construction. There are geographically defined microstates such as Vatican City, with a permanent population measured in the hundreds; there are nations coterminous with archipelagos consisting of hundreds of islands (such as Indonesia); there are nations of mostly contiguous and enormous land masses (Canada, for example). And there are oddities and quirks that lend a rich complexity to our world – one such oddity, defying a 'rational' outlook, is the enclave. An enclave arises when some of the territory of a nation is landlocked within another. A visitor from Vulcan might say: 'Just roll that territory into the larger territory it's surrounded by. It'll be far more convenient, sensible and rational.' The visitor might be surprised to discover that's not at all how humans think about their world: it's not about convenience, it's about loyalties dwelling in imagination. These enclaves are territories within the border of one country which are under the sovereign control of the other country. In Europe, Büsingen am Hochrhein is German, though it is completely surrounded by Swiss territory;[10] border controls were removed in 1967, but getting there involves traversing Swiss territory. Very dramatically, there are enclaves, counter-enclaves and counter-counter-enclaves along the Indian–Bangladeshi border.[11] Individuals within these enclaves lacked the paperwork that would render them not just members of the nation, but recognised as citizens of the state, with the freedoms and papers that being a citizen entails.

It took decades to finally settle this complex situation,[12] with land swaps, and citizens being given the option to choose one nation or the other.

If we were all suddenly afflicted with a peculiar semantic amnesia, one that voided our memories of factual knowledge, our knowledge of borders, of the social, legal and political boundaries we jointly and collectively maintain, then of course these problems would disappear (although the physical installations marking boundaries between nations would not disappear – at least not until nature removed them). And why would you maintain complex border infrastructure, for a social, legal and political purpose (exclusion and control) you can't recall? And how would you maintain a border infrastructure if you are unable to remember how to maintain it? Of course, semantic amnesia is not a viable solution for border disputes, and these border problems will, inevitably, continue to arise.[13]

*

How do we get from shared forms of social organisation such as tribes, clubs and institutions all the way to the formation of nations? The Czech-American political theorist Karl Deutsch (1912–92) was clear in his view of what formed a nation: 'A nation is a group of people united by a mistaken view of their past and hostility toward their neighbors.' That is a sardonic view of nationhood, no doubt, but one reflecting collective mental time travel – particularly to the past – and group identity, predicated on a separateness and comparative antagonism between neighbours.

Here I want to ignore larger national foundation stories arising from history, politics and 'great men'. Instead, let's start with a simple truism: nations are composed of individuals, and, a little more abstractly, nations also comprise our relationships with each other, and our relationships to a particular place and time. Thus our nations consist of individual persons, with all the collective memories and collective understanding such an individually interlocking psychological underpinning implies. And underpinning these are innumerable conversations to align thinking and remembering and acting by those who hold to the common vision of the nation that is or is to be. This is not an inevitable process: some attempts at nation building succeed, some fail, only to be tried again, or just become lost to history.

It was Sir Frederic Bartlett who introduced the concept of 'schema' into the study of memory – the idea that we don't remember the fine details of events, that instead what we do is hang information on to pre-existing knowledge structures which make the recall of such information easier. We can think of collective memory as a schema for organising the story of a people – the guiding narratives of a perhaps mythic or heroic past widely shared among the population.[14] This also makes the telling and retelling of narratives in a simplified but readily transmissible form much easier. Now clearly there is room for difference with respect to the organising schemas, so we can add another category: the reshaping of the narratives of the past. Here collective memory and conversation, identity and imagination intersect.

We can elaborate this idea further. Humans spontaneously organise themselves into groups – through conversation: you must talk first, to get to know someone, in order to decide if they are to be friend or foe. These groups can be very large, and often coalesce around formal and informal institutions (churches, schools, the military). Nations are built on pre-extant interlocking formal and informal institutions. These formal and informal institutions in turn can coagulate into complex and ever-changing, extended hierarchical and heterarchical cognitive structures with interlocking fealties and loyalties and with fused personal and impersonal identities. One telling example is the legal system of a country, which usually includes formal institutions such as courts and laws, and is supported by informal institutions such as social norms and customs. These institutions interact with each other – because of the conversations and decisions the members of these institutions have and make – and shape the country's political and social structure. Legal systems often have peculiar and arbitrary origins, they evolve over time[15] and they become locked-in features of a nation. They show 'path dependency'[16] – a particular outcome arises because of the specific sequence of events and choices that preceded it. Common law and civil law systems are an example. In countries with a common law tradition, like the United States, Ireland and the United Kingdom, the development of laws is based in part on previous court decisions and precedents. Countries with a civil law tradition, like France, have legal systems based on written codes and statutes, and court decisions and precedents play a smaller role in shaping the legal system.

Conversations – in their broadest sense, including media – are used to develop widely shared agreement on what and who comprises the 'nation', aligning memories of all those who share the vision of the nation. This implies that agreement must be established regarding foundational issues of the nation, especially where 'our land' stops and 'your land' starts – the boundaries to the nation must be established, agreed and generally known. There must be a shared, cognitive understanding across individuals where there is a common alignment of knowledge structures among those who regard themselves as members of the nation.

This widespread process of cognitive alignment involves other mental processes, including collective mental time travel – to reinterpret a shared past or agree upon a possible future. Political theorists have long recognised this, even if they do not use this specific framing and language. The influential political theorist Edmund Burke (1729–97),[17] the Irish-born and -raised scion of a Dublin Anglo-Norman family, suggested in his famous work *Reflections on the French Revolution* that society is 'a partnership not only between those who are living, but between those who are living, those who are dead, and those who are to be born'. There are strong echoes of mental time travel here, with references to the past (the dead), the present (those alive) and the future (those yet to be born). Nationhood must exist within a framework of mental time travel – a struggle to exist in the past, a present which could be better, and a glorious future which may yet come to pass; thus collective remembering and shared reality must support this national mental time travel framework. Without memory and imagination to create a shared reality, a nation simply could not exist.

Influenced by Burke, the late and renowned Anglo-Irish political scientist Benedict Anderson,[18] in his deeply influential – and perhaps utterly dominant – analysis of nations as 'imagined communities',[19] asserts that the cornerstone of claims to nationhood, indeed the core of the very concept of nationhood itself, is the idea that we all, as individuals, see ourselves as part of a 'larger imagined community'. Only certain people can vote in national elections (the members of the community) and others cannot (those without the community). National symbols and symbols of national identity, such as flags, anthems and national monuments, are used to create a sense of belonging and shared history among citizens and to remind individuals of their connection to their nation and its people. National holidays and celebrations are used to bring people together and to create a sense of unity and shared identity. (Bastille Day, Independence Day/July the 4th and St Patrick's Day are especially widely recognised, the last celebrated worldwide among the Irish diaspora.) These events often involve rituals and traditions that are specifically designed to evoke feelings of national pride and to remind people of the shared history and values that define their nation. Seeing ourselves as part of a particular imagined community means we imagine that we share certain characteristics and traits setting us apart from other nations. Thus nationhood is essentially a *psychological* concept – one drawing on our inherent human psychological capacities – just as much as nationhood is a legal, political, sociological or indeed historical concept.

Acknowledging these underpinning psychological dimensions, we can understand a nation as an 'imagined political community – and imagined as both inherently limited and sovereign'.[20] The nation is imagined in the sense that other members of the nation live in the mind – because the population of our nation is so much greater than our capacity to meaningfully meet and converse with all those other members. What is missing in Anderson's account is what gets the ball rolling in the first place. You need to be able to imagine alternative futures, you need to be able to travel backwards and forwards on a mental timeline; you need to be able to articulate what you think, have your thoughts tested in conversation, during arguments, in the course of set-piece events: what is missing in Anderson's analysis is a psychologically and neurally plausible account of what drives nation building. I am suggesting here that the first public step in the evolution of any nation is a conversation – one that treats seriously an idea formed in the imagination and then articulated to others along the lines that 'This plot, area, lake, shore-line, territory, field, prairie, land is ours, and we, this family, this tribe, this community, this coalition, will defend it, tend to it, and keep it. And we alone have title to it – no others, and we will pass this land on to our children.' These conversations – in the deep past, before scribes and writing – have not left fossil evidence behind, but nonetheless they must have happened, for articulating to each other goals and plans and intentions sets the stage for everything else that follows.

Conversations of the following type have occurred all over the world:

A furtive meeting, arranged in the corner of a dimly lit room.

Ruritanian revolutionary: 'Comrade, I come to meet with you today to discuss a vision of a united Ruritania and Lower Slobbovia. A new, united nation where our people live in harmony, freed from the shackles of our foreign oppressors. We have so much in common: for our struggles are your struggles, as are our aspirations, and our desires for a better life.'

Lower Slobbovian revolutionary: 'I agree, my friend. We have suffered long under our oppressive rulers. We too dream of a nation where all are treated with dignity and respect. A nation where we can build a just and prosperous society for all.'

Ruritanian revolutionary: 'Exactly! Together we can create a nation where our voices will be heard and our rights protected. A nation where our children grow up in a world of opportunity, not oppression.'

Lower Slobbovian revolutionary: 'We must speak to our peoples, to the peoples of Ruritania and Lower Slobbovia, so they too can be a part of our great dream.'

Ruritanian revolutionary: 'We are not alone, we are many. We shall work together to make this nation a reality.'

Lower Slobbovian revolutionary: 'Yes, we shall make this new nation happen; we will build a better future together.'

(Reader, they do not make this new nation happen.)

But a great politician can speak to all of the nation, perhaps getting a plurality or a majority to adopt a story or narrative that effectively combines thought, action and feeling in the service of the 'imagined community'. There are many such examples. For the American nation, John F. Kennedy, the 35th President of the United States, in his famous inaugural address, called on Americans to 'ask not what your country can do for you – ask what you can do for your country'. This message, emphasising the importance of public service and national unity, helped to galvanise the nation behind Kennedy's leadership. For France, Charles de Gaulle's famous radio broadcasts voiced the spirit of resistance that would see France through the Second World War, famously saying 'Quoi qu'il arrive, la flamme de la résistance française ne doit pas s'éteindre et ne s'éteindra pas' ('Whatever happens, the flame of the French resistance must not and will not be extinguished').[21]

Nations share other characteristics. They are limited in geographic extent, because beyond them are other nations; they are sovereign because the imagined community exercises a right to self-determination within its own territory. They comprise a community because the nation offers a 'deep, horizontal comradeship',[22] with relationships of depth and breadth in thought, action and feeling denied to non-members. This is not to say that territories and nations are uncontested (of course they can be, and often are, contested: boundary disputes are an especially potent source of conflict, but they can be resolved peacefully). And even within a nation there can be multiple, competing visions of the future nation.

Thus nationalism is fundamentally a cognitive project, dependent on an aligning of particular and crucial cognitive constructs across the greater mass of people within a territory. The underlying cognitive processes rely on the senses (we must know how many people live within the nation's boundaries), the map (we must know the extent of the nation's boundaries) and the museum (we must have a sense of the history or the imagined history of the nation). These are the complex 'processes by which the nation came to be imagined and, once imagined, modelled, adapted and transformed'.[23]

Maps and mapping are essential to the nationalist imagination: a nation must have a territory, and that territory is bounded in space and has been established over time. Maps and mapping are, in essence, cognitive exercises, dependent on brain structures that process metrics for space – movement, extent, directions and boundedness, the core components of the cognitive mapping system, involving widespread brain networks embracing the pivotal structures of the hippocampus and anterior thalamus. Recall that damage to these structures (the hippocampus – Henry Molaison;

anterior thalamus – Korsakoff's syndrome) gives rise to a dense and enduring amnesia, with all that that entails for remembering and forgetting. And these structures in turn are co-opted for other uses: in particular, defining boundaries and borders to a territory, and remembering the salient events that have occurred within that territory. Delineating, possessing and controlling territory allow you to define yourself against what occurs in another territory – we (the collective we) are different to them. Notions of time also play a vitally important role in nationhood foundation stories. Mental time travel is vital for the creation and sustenance of newly emerging nations. Specifically, such nations imagine themselves as antique – as old, pre-existing, if only in the imagination – and being old confers legitimacy on claims of nationhood. The members of the nation must also individually and collectively engage in mental time travel to imagine all the tomorrows of the nation's life.

Theorising about time and space makes nationalism a cognitive project, a project requiring a substantial shared or collective memory. A shared sense of nationhood depends on a substantial, shared and stable narrative reaching into the past, but one which also projects forward into a more glorious and fulfilling future. Of course, the contrary impulse might be present – to deny the claims of nationhood simply by denying the antiquity, geography and shared reality at the core of the imagined community.

The idea of nationhood – of belonging to a nation, of citizenship of a nation, among perhaps millions of individuals who do not, and cannot ever, know each other – is almost magical. All of those people identify with each other and are willing to sacrifice for each other, in the name of something which is entirely abstract and intangible. Short of magic spells, though, the idea of nationhood can only arise because we are socialised into a common, cognitive endeavour: an endeavour bringing together memory, imagination and conversation to construct a shared reality at scale. The consequence is to bind us cooperatively, cognitively and affectively together, shaping our very identities. These collective narratives – the stories that come to bind us – organise and outline the temporal and spatial extent of the nation, and help us decide those who are, or can become, members of the nation. And, crucially, these narratives are repeated and retold within and between the generations, giving rise to the continuity required through time for a nation to exist at all.

At an individual level, the stories, tales, songs of the nation – when told and retold – result in synchronisation of brain activity across many individuals simultaneously (and with a very high degree of inter-subject similarity). At an international sporting contest, with fans singing aloud, the brains of all the individuals singing aloud, and indeed of those listening in, become synchronised by the singing of the anthem, telling its tale of the heroic past and glorious future, while offering the chance on the playing field of conquering the opposing side. These are not idle speculations: people sharing the same culture imagine highly similar narratives when listening to the same musical excerpts, whereas those from a dissimilar culture do not.[24]

*

The emergence of nations, in the modern sense, required several key developments, in Anderson's telling. It required the loss of scriptural language and biblical texts as the basis for temporal authority; it required the continued erosion of the divine right of kings to assume power because of birth; and finally, it relied on demerging cosmology and history. Ironically, of course, it was the monk Copernicus who pulled on the thread that eventually sundered the relations of divine scripture, divine blood and divine knowledge. And the church fathers knew how dangerous these new forms of knowledge and learning were for their political–religious project. If God and the earth were no longer at the centre of the cosmos, where did that leave their authority? In tatters has become the answer over the succeeding centuries.

These three forces coming together led to a 'search for a new way of linking fraternity, power and time meaningfully together',[25] a process turbocharged by a new cognitive artefact – the book. One hundred and fifty years or so after the emergence of the printing press there were at least 200 million copies of books in circulation in Europe, for a population of about 78 million people, many of whom could not read. The free circulation of ideas implied by the free circulation of the book – any book – meant that learning and access to ideas were no longer controlled by a church. Books, as extended cognitive artefacts, offloaded memory of facts and events from the brains of individuals, and allowed these memories to be freely available to alter the thoughts, memories, behaviour and allegiances of others. Books are vehicles for stories: the great Irish poet W. B. Yeats believed that there was 'no literature without nationality and no nationality without literature'.[26] Little wonder that book burning and censorship have been supported by authoritarians through the years, for the control of books means the control of ideas.

After the advent of the book, we no longer needed to rely on in-person testimony: we could go and learn something by looking it up ourselves. This allows us to overcome the inherent dangers in our all-too-human bias of 'trusting what we're told'. The remarkable thing is how quickly, over the space of a few centuries, we have come to accept this as an entirely normal, indeed desirable, situation. We now devote enormous amounts of time, money and effort to ensuring universal literacy. Moreover, denying access to education, thereby preventing literacy, is a very effective way of controlling, directing and oppressing a segment of a population, as the terrible and morally repugnant example of contemporary Afghanistan shows us, where an authoritarian and regressive regime is trying to prevent girls from accessing education.

Reading is cognitively demanding, requiring a substantial amount of time and effort on the part of the education system, and of parents or caregivers, to ensure that a child learns how to read. Of course, political regimes all over the world have understood how the education system can in turn be used to shape the collective memory and narrative of a nation by controlling the teaching that goes on within schools. There are numerous examples of this, but a particularly obvious historical one is Nazi Germany, which used the education system to shape the narrative of the nation by controlling the content of textbooks, curriculum and teacher training. The Nazi regime required teachers to teach Nazi ideology to students and promote a particular version of national identity, including crackpot ideas revolving around 'race science'.[27]

Noting the existence of supranational organisations, Anderson suggested that we will be willing to die for the imagined and shared communities of our nations, but we will not die for the organisations our nations are part of. This consideration was written in 1983 when Comecon (the Soviet bloc's Council for Mutual Economic Assistance – 1949–91) existed. Within a few years, Comecon had disappeared, and nobody died trying to preserve it. The EEC (European Economic Community – 1957–2009), as was, no longer exists, having transformed itself into the European Union, an unusual international treaty organisation. EU member states bind themselves together through cognitive artefacts – treaties – to jointly protect their interests in the world at large, by changing how the nation states comprising the EU themselves function.[28] And, of course, soldiers do fight and die as part of international alliances and coalitions (such as NATO, or when on UN peacekeeping operations).

Countries have come and gone since Anderson wrote those words: in Europe, the German Democratic Republic (7 October 1949–3 October 1990) disappeared, and Germany was reunited; Czechoslovakia dissolved itself into two countries, the Czech Republic, or Czechia, and Slovakia. One listing suggests that thirty-four countries have come into existence since 1990, with South

Sudan as the most recent new nation achieving recognition;[29] other countries may disappear, split or be reorganised substantially in the coming decades. Which nations may come or go is difficult to predict, but it can be predicted that as new ones emerge, calls to an ancient claim of nationhood will be made, coupled with visions of a wonderful future – the land of 'milk and honey' will make an appearance. Appeals will be made to shared and exclusive identity – inclusive of some, and against others. These appeals are necessarily appeals to memory and imagination, as we shall see next.

9.
IMAGINING OUR FUTURE NATIONS, TOGETHER

We set off on the unlikely road we have taken thus far by focusing on the price we pay as individuals when our memories fail us – for ourselves and for our network of relationships with others. We then considered the networks of relationships between language use, memory and our intense social lives, and how we use memory and language to create shared social worlds. I've described a new way of thinking about human memory – thinking of it as being at the core of social communication, allowing us to remember and know things together, to construct shared mental realities, particularly through the conversations we have together. Memory is central to enabling us to construct shared cognitive realities, ranging in scale from couples to the imagined entities that are our nations. The intensive focus on memory as a personal phenomenon – one situated in the heads of individuals – causes us to miss these larger perspectives.

The nations of the world are cognitively arbitrary ways through which we carve up our imagined communities into manageable entities, a contention that opens up many important questions. Why do people feel such attachment to this invention of their shared imaginations, and why are people willing to die for this invention? What will be the future of any particular nation? How stable are nations? Will any nation survive indefinitely, or will it eventually dissolve or break into more manageable constituent parts if there is a loss of commitment to a unifying national story? What happens to a nation if orthodoxy requires an unyielding loyalty to a single interpretation of the nation (perhaps promulgated by a 'Great Leader'), and if its citizens slowly decouple themselves from this interpretation, offering only surface compliance? The philosopher Daniel Dennett uses the metaphor of 'universal acid' to describe how new ideas can change or challenge existing beliefs and understanding and how they can 'eat through' or dissolve other ideas or concepts.[1] Does this widespread individual hypocrisy gradually congeal into something more like a universal acid dissolving the institutions that bind the nation together?

Other disciplines might provide potential answers regarding the formation of nations at other levels of analysis. Explanations from political science for the formation of nations tend to focus on the role of the state and political processes (such as the creation of a shared sense of identity and the emergence of a centralised government). History, as a discipline, generally focuses on the role of historical events, such as wars or colonialism, in shaping national identity. Economic explanations focus on the role of economic factors, such as the development of trade or the growth of industry. Anthropological explanations focus on culture (such as shared language, religion or customs. A sociobiologist – someone who analyses and examines social behaviour in terms of evolution – might, for example, suggest that this willingness arises from shared kinship, and hence from an instinct for preservation of genes. Truth be told, this level of analysis is not helpful given our current state of knowledge. There is no demonstrable relationship between the genomics of kinship and the formation of nationhood. Moreover, even handwaving in the direction of genetics as a meaningful basis for nationhood falters in the face of the creation and relentless growth of the United States of America, the immigrant nation with transfusions of unrelated people from all over the globe, who live together in a relative state of harmony. In New York City alone, there are at least 700 languages spoken other than English;[2] the USA is not alone in achieving these levels of peaceful integration of diverse populations. Many other countries have absorbed proportionately very large immigrant populations over the past hundreds of years. My own country, Ireland, for example, now has an estimated foreign-born population of approximately 17% of its residents – it was only a few percent two generations ago. The vast urban agglomeration that is London has a foreign-born population of approximately 37%,[3] again living in relative harmony. In fact, paradoxically, the highest rates of acceptance of immigrants tend to be in the places where there are the greatest degree of contact between the native population and immigrants, whereas resentment against immigrants tends to be highest in places where they are fewest in number. Mere exposure to others creates the immediate possibility of affiliation and attachment to others.

Charles Darwin, perhaps echoing Burke's influence a little, remarked in his book *The Descent of Man* (1871) that there 'can be no doubt that a tribe including many members who, from possessing in a high degree the spirit of patriotism, fidelity, obedience, courage, and sympathy, were always ready to aid one another, and to sacrifice themselves for the common good, would be victorious over most other tribes; and this would be natural selection'.[4] One of the most potent forces in the creation of nations is nationalism – the sense shared among people of a particular place and time that 'this is our nation, and we are loyal to it; we are devoted to it; and we have the right to self-determination over ourselves'. We need to think more seriously about a psychological framework for understanding nationalism; it has not really been a topic treated as a mainstream psychological phenomenon, despite nationalism being perhaps the major organising principle of our larger political lives. It has been treated more as a political, sociological and historical phenomenon. Pulling together the elements of the framework elaborated through this book, and adding some add-itional concepts, we arrive at the following contention: nationalism of any particular type is learned through exposure to, and immer-sion in, a particular culture; we are ready from early life to absorb nationalist ideologies.

Our capacity for nationalism arises from the common biology of interactions between many different brains drawing on shared capacities to remember and imagine things afresh together in story-telling and conversation. Nationalism is a potent psychological force, addressing a laundry list of psychological needs and leverag-ing others. It provides a means of affiliation and identification with others and crucially with their shared, abstract, imaginative goals, as well as participation in shared endeavours – and thus is a means of engaging in social and parasocial relationships. National-ism offers a cognitive shortcut to define membership of in-groups (the nation) and out-groups (all the other nations); membership of particular in-groups brings numerous social rewards, as well as potential resource allocation and resource sharing (one of the canonical tales of nation building is how status, ranks and resources are bundled and parcelled out). During the nation-building pro-cess in the United States, for example, land was a key resource parcelled out to individuals and groups through a system of land grants, homesteads and land purchases. Status and rank were also important factors in the distribution of resources, with wealthy and influential individuals often receiving preferential treatment. And this process involved appropriation of the land of Native Americans, who were regarded as less than worthy of equal treat-ment and rights. On the other side of the world, a similar process was underway: the Treaty of Waitangi, signed in 1840, established a formal relationship between the British Crown and the indigen-ous Māori people of New Zealand. It granted the Māori certain rights and protections, but also granted the Crown the right to govern and make laws for the country. This treaty established a hierarchy in which the British had a higher status and more resources, while the Māori were granted certain rights and privileges. These are not singular examples: history books are replete with similar accounts through the millennia.

Nationalist movements can offer routes to power, a means of dominating others and engaging in corrupt resource extraction, either personally or facilitating it by others. The signal example of Adolf Hitler almost a century ago, and the more recent example of Slobodan Milošević (on a smaller scale), show that fomenting hatreds through nationalism and anti-Semitism are effective vehicles for attaining such dark and destructive power. However, nationalism can also offer a way to attain status through service to others. Some obvious examples of the latter are Mahatma Gandhi and Nelson Mandela, both devoted to their nations and their peoples, and leaving a posthumous legacy of how to attain status through service to others. Gandhi, widely revered as the father of modern India, gave an especially powerful example as leader of India's independence movement, using non-violent civil disobedience to peacefully resist British rule. I visited his memorial in Raj Ghat in Delhi while on a trip to India – a country I love to visit – and was awestruck by the numbers attending, the strange stillness in the air preserving the shape of the beautiful flower rangoli on his tomb, and the reverence of the crowd present.

We are cognitive misers, and want to minimise unnecessary expenditure of energy (thinking is hard, after all; swift judgements are much easier, bypassing the need for considered judgement). Nationalism provides an identity lens to see the world through (simplifying the world), as well as a handy guide to the imagination of the cognitive world of the individual, by leveraging shared concepts and language ('sea to shining sea'; 'government of the people, by the people, for the people, shall not perish from the earth'). Thus nationalism is a way to order one's place in the world; and a way to exert some control (at least through understanding) of the world. Nationalism can bring with it a strong sense of inclusivity and exclusivity, with an immediate reading through to perceived status (hence the rankings of passports). In consequence, it offers a means of envisioning others, so that the members of one nation can ask, rightly or wrongly, of another: does the other nation have a right to exist? Do we see its existence as legitimate, or as a threat to us? Is it a mere plaything to be taken back under a war of colonial conquest? These are not idle questions: when people deny agency – the ability to make decisions and choices – to the citizens of other nations because of their own limited, nationalistic perspective, this can be a prime cause of conflict. Indigenous peoples in colonised countries have often been denied agency and treated as inferiors, with potent prejudices expressed regarding their dignity, equality and worth as human beings. This naturally has led to ongoing conflicts and injustices, as their basic rights and autonomy are not recognised by those in power. More recently, the invasion of Ukraine by Russia seems to have been conceived in similar terms: a denial of Ukraine's right to exist, the right to have its borders respected, and the right of the citizens of Ukraine to make their own decisions. The citizens of other nations obviously also possess their own nationalist imagination, and potently so under threat, for the dangerous out-group is brought into stark relief.

Nationalism as a shared cognitive project provides what seems like a way to participate in defining the future path of the nation. The possibilities for the future seem endless – nationalism thus invokes an expansive and collective sense of mental time travel, fantasising (in the parochial sense of imaginative thinking, disconnected from the here and now) about visions of a glorious future contrasted with an ignoble past. It therefore offers a strange form of immortality – participatory and collective, cleaving to a common vision of the future of the nation. We remember our nationalist heroes, putting them on pedestals, naming streets after them, invoking them on days of national celebration.

Nationalism will usually beat a technocratic vision of the

future, because it leverages potent, immediate, fast-responding psychological processes. Technocracy promises things will slowly and incrementally get better, with a promise of, say, a 2% annual improvement in living standards, leading them to double every two generations.[5] Two salient examples of consequential technocrats are, respectively, Goh Keng Swee of Singapore, and T. K. Whitaker of Ireland, both hugely influential behind-the-scenes figures in similarly populated island economies with large, and occasionally difficult, neighbours. Both Swee and Whitaker devised and implemented policies aimed at increasing education and developing infrastructure and technology to transform their nations into prosperous and diversified export-oriented economies. Both technocrats' efforts demonstrate the potential for economic technocracies to improve a nation's economic situation through sustainable, long-term policies. Yet who has heard of these two? I suspect few enough within their own countries, and neither is a nationalist icon. Yet the living standards of their countries are measurably and substantially better for their work.

Nationalism bypasses a central psychological bias against piecemeal progress; we are better at seeing categorical progress, and overlook positive, piecemeal, incremental progress. When it comes to progress, people tend to 'lump' things together. When entities make efforts to improve, people tend to dismiss them if they don't achieve complete reform. This is because falling short is seen as a lack of commitment to real change. As a result, people tend to undervalue and underinvest in incremental improvements. When efforts to solve a problem fail, people may overlook smaller, but still important, steps that might be taken.[6] The reality is that, in the absence of special training or a pressing need, most of us are not interested in time-series data showing incremental change positively compounding over time. Moreover, a large-scale empirical survey discloses that, compared with what is actually observed in the world, we humans have 'a pervasive tendency, across ideological and demographic categories, to see things as getting worse than they really are"[7] – we do not keep abreast of the latest empirical data, and we don't usually go to empirical sources such 'Our World in Data'[8] to test what we think and to update the empirical contents of our beliefs. And, of course, we are novelty-seeking, and we want the new thing, even if what we want is not what we need: potentially, a new nation, or a new status for the existing nation – a new way of life, a fresh start, a better future.

Further answers regarding attachment to the nation might be found by exploring the blending of individual psychological and social processes. The sociologist Émile Durkheim originally proposed that when we gather in a purposive group we can experience 'collective effervescence' – a kind of 'contagious euphoria'.[9] We easily and readily experience a 'psychological high' as part of a crowd gathered for a collective reason – a march, attending a concert, participating in a religious ritual or cheering (or indeed jeering) at a sports match, for example. The feeling of 'effervescent assembly', the individual psychological benefit from participating in group activity, is an important social phenomenon, sustaining group activity and identity. People who feel they are part of a crowd report at least transient increases in their feeling of wellbeing. Collective effervescence has been measured by asking participants to rate statements such as 'I feel connected to others when in a large group activity I like, like going to a concert, church, or a convention,' or 'When I attend a wedding I feel a connection to the other people there.' Scoring more highly tends to correlate with lower levels of self-reported loneliness, higher levels of positive feelings and meaning in life, and feeling more connected with others.[10] One study examined the relative importance of sacred values, moral convictions and identity fusion in respect of gun rights or abortion rights, with endorsement of fighting and dying for the cause as the measure.[11] A combination of the feeling of the defiling of sacred values, violations of one's moral convictions and the fusing of the personal self with a cause (identity fusion) were found at the core of the claimed willingness to sacrifice oneself for a cause. Remarkably, these motivations are among those reported by Turkish citizens who joined ISIS[12] and by foreign fighters in Ukraine.[13] Both cases suggest a blurring of the boundaries between the self and the nation, and a willingness to sacrifice the self in the cause of the nation.

We need to consider plausible psychological mechanisms by which acts of collective remembering and acts of collective imagination come to be shared between individuals to create a shared reality that acts as a guide to the future and not simply the past. We have discussed the work of the Columbia University psychologist Tory Higgins and his colleagues investigating how we come to create shared realities – how we come to believe the same things, and act together on those beliefs.[14] People come to believe the same things and work together; and reality becomes shared when people share with each other their feelings, beliefs and thoughts about the world. The vital part of creating a shared reality is the idea of 'sharing is believing': when people talk to each other, they usually tell each other what they're thinking and feeling, and they usually believe what the other person says. This helps us to be attuned to each other, and build shared institutions and organisations and even the big idea of a nation. To pick up a theme of this book: nations start as conversations. These conversations may between revolutionaries ('we will take this land, and make it a nation': how many countries have begun like this?), or they may be between parliamentarians. But, this where they start: the articulation of a vision for the future nation, by people willing to work to make it happen.

In conversation, we generally reveal ourselves – what we're thinking, what we're feeling – to other individuals quickly and without much of an effort to truly hide what we really feel (unless hiding what we truly think or feel matters in some way, in which case we dissimulate, shape our responses to who we're talking to or straightforwardly lie), and as listeners our default state is generally to believe what the other person says, to assume that they are not deliberately lying to us, that when they tell us what they are thinking that is in fact what they are thinking.

These ideas make sense of what otherwise would be great mysteries regarding our social worlds. Our social world is complex and depends on a considerable degree of unquestioning trust in each other, and we generally recognise that lying, especially by public figures, is corrosive of the public good (unless of course they are *our* public figures – figures with whom we have an intense parasocial relationship, in which case their lying gets them a free pass). After all, what are a few lies between friends, especially when they are for the greater good? Higgins and his colleagues suggest that 'sharing is believing' involves two processes which are synergistic with each other. Sharing is believing leads to increased interpersonal closeness on the one hand, and to an increase in how strongly we believe ('epistemic certainty') on the other. If we believe what the other person is saying, we feel closer to that person and we are more likely to accept the truth of the assertions they make about things.

This co-created reality can go awry at a microlevel within couples, in the rare syndrome known as *folie à deux* (from the French for 'madness for two') – a condition where two individuals share a common delusion, remember it and live it. The Canadian film director David Cronenberg's disturbing and disquieting movie *Dead Ringers* is based on the real-life case of twins who traded identities with each other and seemed to suffer from *folie à deux*. The British actor Jeremy Irons played both twins, named Elliot and Beverly Mantle in the movie. At one point, underscoring the extreme identification and co-dependency the twins have developed with each other, Eliot says, 'Why are you crying, Bev?', and Beverly replies, 'Separation can be a . . . terrifying thing.' Separation means a sundering of their fused identity, of their shared lives, of their joint cognitive and emotional realities. Eliot and Beverly fall into a shared delusion fuelled by drug dependency, eventually leading to their deaths.

This condition also goes by more modern names such as 'shared psychotic disorder', 'induced delusional disorder', 'shared psychosis' and 'shared delusional disorder'. The condition was originally described formally in 1877 by Charles Lasègue and Jules Falret (and is sometimes called Lasègue–Falret syndrome). The core of *folie à deux* is a shared, co-dependent, delusional system, sustained and supported by mutually reinforcing conversation. For a diagnosis of *folie à deux*, the partners must be intimately associated; there must be a similarity in the content of their delusional beliefs; further, the couple involved must each accept, share and support the delusions that are expressed by the other. I am tempted by the idea that there is a generalised form of *folie à deux* that occasionally infects polities and political parties, where a clearly crazy idea spreads among individuals, who find themselves saying and identifying with political, economic and other positions that to an outsider look utterly detached from empirical reality.

Because psychiatric disorders are best understood as being on a spectrum, rather than as a categorical all-or-nothing condition – you either have one or you don't – the sharing of somewhat delusionary beliefs may happen more frequently but in a less pathological form, or even a non-pathological form, in the population at large. One person in a couple might come, for example, to share the other's obsessions with the prophetic powers of newspaper horoscopes, support their partner in this belief and even come to profess some belief in them. And pushing beyond this, a kind of *folie de la société* might exist to a greater degree than anyone cares to admit. Wealth, for example, is a shared, cognitive construct – one we choose to believe in. And when we believe too much, we get 'tulip fever'; we start to believe that 'this time, it's different',[15] that house prices can only go up (until they don't); and when we stop believing, we get an Enron . . .

Two important primary human motivations intersect here: the need to connect with others, and the need to understand and comprehend the world. We want to share 'reality', meaning we shape what we say according to how we read the needs and attitudes and beliefs of the other person. The extent to which these are congruent and mutually rewarding corresponds to the extent to which we 'click' or not with others. Beliefs about the world and about how we should behave within the world, of course, can form a hierarchy where superordinate beliefs trump subordinate beliefs. Beliefs about respect for others, for example, can be hierarchical, where the superordinate belief of respect for others trumps subordinate beliefs, such as speaking without considering others' feelings, or prioritising our own needs above others. In other words, respect for others is recognised as more important than conflicting personal desires or beliefs. I've previously mentioned Gandhi: he believed in the principles of *satya* (truth) and *ahimsa* (nonviolence), and led nonviolent protests and boycotts. He remained committed to nonviolence and respect for others, despite facing persecution from the British authorities, when a campaign of violence might have been an easier response. In a differing example, scientists are generally motivated to try to understand the world, but can and do vigorously disagree with each other (as anyone who has been through the rigours of peer review will attest).[16] Paradoxically, scientists may feel closer to each other, despite their disagreement, because disagreements are generally data-driven and data-led, because the identity lens through which they view the world is evidence-based.

*

Is it possible for individuals to engage in *national* mental time travel?[17] The starting point here is the idea that politicians, in their set-piece speeches, evoke memories of the past to shape the image their public forms of the future. Sigmund Freud expressed it thus: 'Words have magical power. They can transfer knowledge from teacher to student; words enable the orator to sway his audience and dictate its decisions. Words are capable of arousing the strongest emotions and prompting all men's actions.'[18] The orator's imaginative invocation of the future happens in the present, drawing on the imagination and memory of those listening.

The historic events shaping a nation might not be 'personally experienced', even for major events that could be hugely consequential. There is an important difference between being there at the event and hearing about it through news media. The example of 9/11 is often used. In relative terms, few people directly experienced or witnessed 9/11. Most people experienced that day's horrors mediated through news channels of one description or another, rather than being present at, for example, the site of the Twin Towers in New York. The most you can do is imagine yourself standing looking at the morning sky at 8.30 a.m. Eastern Time in New York on 11 September 2001, a morning like any other sunny, clear September morning, going about your day. By 9.30 a.m., the course of history had been rewritten in an instant, with the murderous attack perpetrated by Al Qaeda. We are living with the transnational consequences of that day still.

Individuals participating in groups might try to imagine the future, and they do so jointly – perhaps most explicitly through conversation. Individuals, even isolated individuals, employ memories of a collective past to imagine a collective future. Because we share, to some degree within the one community, memories of our past, these elements of our remembering in some way might enter our imagining of a collective future. There are, of course, some problems with this way of thinking. It has consistently been found that people, when surveyed, are more positive about their own personal future than they are about their nation's future. Similarly, when asked to look back on their lives, people show a marked 'positivity bias' where they recall more positive things compared to the 'negativity bias' they show when recalling their nation's past. These elements, therefore, can markedly complicate the nature of collective mental time travel when imagining one's own nation's future compared to imagining one's own personal future.

The psychologists Meymune Topcu and William Hirst of the

New School for Social Research, New York, set out to explore several factors in relation to the imagining of the nation's future by individuals.[19] They asked participants to remember fifteen events over the past fifty years and to imagine fifteen events that might occur over the next fifty years (with ratings).[20] This is not an easy task, is it? Finally, they also asked participants to rate the 'entitativity' of the item in question. Entitativity refers to the group's perceived unity and cohesiveness. This is based on the group's shared characteristics, history, goals and outcomes. In other words, entitativity measures the extent to which the group sees itself as having a unified purpose and agency in its actions The idea, essentially, is to focus on the coherence of the action or actions of the group as a whole.

Topcu and Hirst grouped the categories their participants used to think about past and future events.[21] These were: violence/terrorism, the environment, finance, political legislative, political/parties, political international, war/military, human rights, sports, cultural, science and technology/space, health, energy and other. People did not extend themselves so terribly far into the past. Over the two experiments, people remembered back between seventeen and a half and nineteen years on average. Imagining the future showed a degree of 'temporal compression', where time appears more condensed or squashed: on average, people imagined events between eleven and thirteen years hence. Seemingly, we can remember somewhat further back in time than we can imagine forward in time.

One important finding in this work is related to the degree of personal versus impersonal agency that individuals felt. By and large, people believe that the agents that have affected the past or can affect the future are non-persons – they are institutions and organisations. These non-persons were regarded as affecting the course of the past on about 60% of occasions, and of the future on about 75% of occasions. Interestingly, people have an agency bias towards the future, both for themselves and for their nation. That is to say, they believe that the nation would be able to do more things in the future than it was possible for it to have done in the past.

Partisan political identity is the strength of one's affiliation to a particular political cause – the extent, for example, to which you strongly identify as a MAGA-nation/America First person, or a Kentuckian, or . . . (if you're an American; you can create this list for any nation you choose). Surprisingly, it appears that partisan political identity does not enter into people's imagining of their own personal future or into their imagining of the nation at large. This is perhaps a heartening outcome, because partisan political identity does not seem to markedly distort the average person's thinking about the future. For most people who are not deeply politically involved, their political identity may be a means of providing social connection more than anything else, where individuals take low-effort actions to signal support cost-free for a cause (liking preferred causes on Twitter or Facebook, for example). Political identity may serve as a way to signal membership of a social group or express independence rather than representing a strongly held belief or commitment to a cause.

Thinking about the future inevitably draws upon our memory of our past experiences,[22] because there is a strong relationship between how people remember their past and how they imagine their own personal, individual future. This is also true for their country: there is a strong relationship between how people remember their country's past and how they imagine their country's future. Thus if it is the case that there are national memories, then national future thinking (prospection) should be strongly related to those memories, and this is indeed what Topcu and Hirst found. Participants were more likely to 'imagine specifically phenomenally rich and positive future events if their memories of past national events had corresponding levels of these attributes'.[23] A remarkable and enduring example is the United States' Declaration of Independence, and the founding principles of life, liberty and the pursuit of happiness. These foundational memories have influenced the country's collective prospection, or thinking about its future, by shaping its values and guiding its actions as a nation. The moonshot, President Kennedy's challenge to put a man on the moon, was an historic and memorable moment of national pride and achievement in the US. If the United States continues to remember the moonshot as such a moment, it may be motivated to set ambitious goals for the future, such as sending humans to Mars (as Elon Musk dreams) or developing new technologies that have the potential to revolutionise society.

Mentally travelling forward in time allows for more agency than travelling back in time, but mentally travelling forward doesn't go as far into the future as mentally travelling into the past. The roads not yet travelled have yet to be chosen, and agency manifests itself in the choices that you know you have yet to make. Paradoxically, here we have one of the failures that might occur in human imagination. Changes that occur over longer timescales are difficult for us to imagine and therefore perhaps more difficult for us to take seriously. Perhaps the great difficulty we have in dealing with climate change is that the changes occurring are slow and imperceptible and play out on timescales that extend beyond individual human lives. Climate change seems to be like bankruptcy: it happens 'gradually, then suddenly'.[24] Training future-oriented cognition to deal with these kinds of issues may therefore require us to engage in 'intergenerational imagination', where we must try to imagine outcomes whereby our children or our grandchildren deal with the problems that climate change will present over a fifty- or hundred-year timescale.

Our understanding of how the brain participates in, or supports, collective memory has hardly started as an area of investigation. Much more progress has been made in understanding collective memory as a psychological or cultural phenomenon. There are some important clues, though, regarding how collective memory might be represented within the brain. A particular region of the frontal lobes of the brain – known as the prefrontal cortex – is likely to be implicated. This brain region is subdivided into the dorsomedial prefrontal cortex (DMPFC), which is towards the top of the skull, and the ventromedial prefrontal cortex (VMPFC), which is closer to the eyeballs. These parts of the prefrontal cortex are regarded as elements of the brain's 'social network', for they are involved intimately in understanding the self and its relation to others and in understanding the experiences of others.[25] For example, these brain areas are particularly active when thinking about what others might believe (social judgement); when considering the pain that another person might be suffering (empathy); or when making judgements about the descriptiveness of individual words applied to oneself or to other people (social description or social classification).

Armed with these insights, Pierre Gagnepain and his colleagues at the University of Caen in France used a combination of archival techniques, brain imaging, behavioural studies of a war memorial and machine learning (a computer program that can learn to 'problem solve' through exposure to data; voice- and face-recognition programmes are a common example) to examine if collectively held memories in France of the Second World War provide schemas predicting the organisation of memories by individuals of that war.[26] It might be the case that the repetitive collective presentation of memories related to the war shape what individuals remember or know of that war. It seems likely that this repetitive presentation should have some effect, but what?

Gagnepain and his colleagues examined thirty years of broadcasts on French television concerning the Second World War, derived from television archives. These broadcasts were converted to text, and analysed to find the consistent main themes on television of information concerning the war. A group of participants was also taken on a guided tour through the French National War Memorial at Caen. These participants then underwent brain imaging while actively remembering images of specific points of interest or particular places at the war memorial site itself. Gagne-pain and his colleagues then examined the relationship between collective memories of the war derived from the television broad-casts and the organisation of individual memory. Collective schemas created by the analysis of television broadcasts more accurately predicted the organisation of individual memories than did models of the content of semantic memory (these are formal models of such content that attempt to explain how the brain rep-resents and organises information about concepts and general knowledge). The schemas from television broadcasts correlated better with brain activity than did models of semantic memory. This seems to vindicate Halbwachs's claim that 'our recollections depend on those of all our fellows and on the great frameworks of the memory of society'.[27] Moreover, 'elements unique to collective memory are in DMPFC'[28] (dorsomedial prefrontal cortex). In summary, Gagnepain and his colleagues say, 'Humans maintain group consistency and identity across space and time (gener-ations) using collective memory, which is permitted by specific cultural tools and means.'

The repetitive presentation of television broadcasts powerfully influences the schemas individuals use to organise and understand important and significant parts of their own national history. This has been understood for generations by advertisers and propagan-dists. Shaping the message and presenting that message repetitively, with slight variations, allows that message to become part of our collective memory. The most important point made by the work of Gagnepain and his colleagues is that there is a locus in the overall memory system of the brain which is especially implicated in col-lective memory. Korsakoff's patients have particular damage to a part of the brain known as the anterior thalamus. The anterior thalamus sends connections to and receives connections from both the dorsal medial and the ventromedial components of the pre-frontal cortex. It is thus a reasonable possibility that Korsakoff's patients, who are known to have deficits in social and emotional memory processing, may also show deficits in collective memory, but this hypothesis has yet to be tested.[29]

*

The historian James Wertsch and the psychologist Roddy Roediger emphasise the importance of distinguishing between collective recall and formal history.[30] Collective recall is essentially a national identity project with associated narratives of heroism by the members of the nation, a harking back to a golden age for society, etc. Collective recall is intolerant of ambiguity and discounts counter-evidence in favour of particularly established narratives, and it involves implicit theories, schemas and scripts that simplify the past and ignore findings that sit outside the narrative. Moreover, it is sticky in quality, it is conservative and resistant to change, and it is present in the popular, rather than the historian's, mind, whereas formal history attempts an objective account of what has happened in the past, even if this results in demands for an updating of the identity of the individual regarding their nation. Formal history is comfortable with complexity and ambiguity; it is revised in the light of new evidence, with narratives that change in response to new information. Thus formal history can be uncomfortable – indeed very challenging – when counterposed to common, general memories of history. I don't claim here that what people are saying to each other is accurate or true. Historians are well used to the phenomenon of contested narratives about events; there is a strong and important sense in which we contest the interpretation of the events of the past because this allows us to contest and possibly capture our possible imagined futures.

Historians who attempt to contest and reshape our general understanding of topics are sometimes referred to as 'revisionists'. Such historians are often figures of controversy, especially if they are seen as individuals who attempt to whitewash or propagandise on behalf of a particular political regime. However, the process of revising narratives does not necessarily depend on the intervention of historians: times move along, the meanings of words shift and our understanding of actions in particular contexts can become very different as generational change occurs and there is a distance in time from the events described. In 2018, French President Emmanuel Macron caused controversy when he said that France bore responsibility for the torture and abuse of Algerian independence fighters during the Algerian War of Independence (1954–62).[31] Macron's comments were described by members of Marine Le Pen's National Rally party as 'yet another sign of weakness' and an attempt to declare a 'memory war' on the people of France and their history.[32] Controversies like this can be found in every nation because of the sensitivity that many politicians feel when it comes to discussing certain historical topics. Every country is prone to outbreaks of contested interpretation of the past, especially in times of difficulty and uncertainty. But memories of colonialism and memories of empire vary dramatically depending on who is telling the story – the conquered and colonised have different tales to tell from those of the conqueror and coloniser. Sadly, the latter are usually the ones who get to dominate the discourse.

History is selectively recounted – especially in conversation. We, the general public, are not professional historians, offering nuanced, archive-sourced, monograph-length recountings of our past. You as an individual experience your own past personally, and in turn imagine your own future individually. You might discuss your own future in and with small social groups such as friends and families. And future planning for children is particularly important in families. Conversation is central to all such future planning, and this conversation is personally experienced. The national conversation does not do nuance: it is a schematised, sometimes bowdlerised, scrappy recounting of the past, generally serving present interests rather than scholarly accuracy and completeness. Politicians, through set-piece speeches and their frequent media appearances, can drive historical understanding in directions that are not historically accurate. These statements about the historical past can reshape people's memories of that past.[33] Our memory is dynamic and reconstructive, and can be, and is, shaped by the conversations we have with others. Selective rememberings and recountings of a shared national history by high-status members of a community, such as politicians, may affect what people remember, especially if the politician is one with whom they have a strong parasocial relationship. This might be amplified by social media – for example, the delivery via Twitter of the seeming inner thoughts of a politician, direct to the screen in your hand on an apparently moment-by-moment basis. The key point here is that remembering is goal-directed. The psychologist Charles Stone and his colleagues suggest that the citizens of a country 'will often frame how they remember its history by having as a goal to remember past events that support their view of their nation'.[34]

The implication, therefore, is that if your view of your nation emphasises particular aspects of your nation's past – strengths or weaknesses, glory or dishonour, helplessness or courage – then the events you recall will be overwhelmingly shaped by the views you hold. This remains true even though the history of any nation will be much more complex and complicated than the schematised events that any one individual recalls as being crucial to their nation: 'History telling is often a means of buttressing social identity.'[35] Napoleon allegedly said, somewhat cynically, that 'History is a set of lies, agreed upon' ('L'histoire est une suite de mensonges sur lesquels on est d'accord').[36] Our personal readings of history are not neutral, for they sculpt our memories. When a particular reading and interpretation of history is undertaken to enhance social bonds, information that would erode those bonds is forgotten, passed over in silence or simply de-emphasised, and other events more strongly amplified. Listening to, watching or reading historical events threatening one's social identity has little chance of become part of a shared collective memory because collective memories reflect important aspects of social identity that do not speak to the complexity of our past as it has occurred.

The account I have provided here is clearly missing out on much that is important. The fusing of religion, politics and nationalism has been one of the most potent forces over the past two millennia, especially in the making and breaking of nations and empires. But some elements can be especially emphasised: the fusing of religion, politics (understood as history in action in the present – agency and common memory as one) and nationalism brings people together with a common story and shared goals; these stories and goals can be transmitted through conversation and storytelling from person to person, aligning them behaviourally, affectively and cognitively. In Ireland, the fusion of religion, politics and nationalism in the late nineteenth and early twentieth centuries brought many people together with a common story and shared goals. For example, the Irish nationalist movement blurred the definition of Irish identity and culture as fundamentally Catholic, and promoted Catholic values and traditions as central to the nation's character. Time and again we see this fusing of religion and nationalism in numerous other countries: in India, for example, with the rise of Hindu nationalism; in the USA, with certain members of Congress explicitly declaring themselves 'Christian nationalists'; or with Iran and Saudi Arabia explicitly proclaiming themselves constitutional theocracies. This fusing would not be so potent if it did not easily draw upon underlying psychological and brain states: nationalism maps to a particular geographical place with defined borders; religion to (eternal) time; politics to action in the here and now (while occasionally holding out hope for the better times to come). Religion, politics and nationalism bring together stories, time and place that make sense of the world and of the place of the person and their community within the world.

Establishing, and binding together, people in an imagined, shared collective can only happen as the result of people learning, reshaping and relearning what they know together – which, in turn, moulds their identity. Our memory allows us to interpret and adapt to the present, and allows us to imagine possible futures. Memory allows us to create a shared, collective social reality: our use of memory in everyday conversation allows us to create shared realities from the threads of our individual and social identities and lives. But our stories of our past are just that: narratives reflecting elements of an identity serving membership of our social groups.

*

Our shared realities are created by brains, but so too are the approximations we make to shared, objective truthful realities using empirical methods: we use our brains to create our understanding of our shared realities, but we also can (and sometimes do) use our brains to systematically collect facts and evidence to understand the truth about the world. Our sensory and cognitive systems are limited, fragile and bounded. Edmund Burke recognised this more than two centuries ago: 'We are afraid to put men to live and trade each on his own private stock of reason; because we suspect that this stock in each man is small, and that the individuals would do better to avail themselves of the general bank and capital of nations and of ages.'[37]

There is much about the world we don't know, and certainly much that we don't know we don't know. But there is an absolute evolutionary constraint: shared beliefs that refuse empirical reality may result in the untimely death of their adherents: one shared belief that refuses empirical reality is the rejection of modern medicine in favour of 'alternative' treatments, which can lead to the untimely death of adherents who have not received proven medical treatments. Just as there might be a lot of ruin in a nation, there is a lot of flexibility in belief systems as long as they do not go against the rules that ensure the survival and reproduction of future generations. You are free to believe all sorts of palpable nonsense, such as aliens controlling our government, so long as they don't result in a Darwin Award. The good news is that there is no real weight of history pressing upon us; there are no years of the past bearing down upon us. There is only our individual and collective memory of that past; there are only the stories we tell about that past; there is only what we learn and carry from the past and present to imagine the future.

What we collectively remember and collectively imagine is necessarily simplified, schematised, storified, narrativised. We, the members of our nations, are not professional historians testing hypotheses and propositions about our nation's past against the contents of the archives. Rather, we learn fitfully and sporadically about the historical past, and we keep this version of the past alive in our social groups in the service of our collective remembering, thereby sustaining our identity and membership of those groups. Understanding the dynamics of these processes points the way to how we can free ourselves from mutual enmity and hatred. Perhaps we should try to collectively remember more, embrace complexity, allow ourselves to imagine alternative futures, and act to forestall future potential disasters, and reach our great potential as the only species on this planet capable of bringing into being a shared, imagined reality. Our capacity to remember together and critically, *to talk about it together*, has fashioned our world – our hypersocial, hypercomplex world, populated by our imaginings and longings, rendered possible by the residue of our malleable memories, shaped and reshaped by the stories we tell each other about ourselves and each other, and our longings for a better, alternative tomorrow. We should demand no less of ourselves and the present moment.

AFTERWORD

This book was conceived in what some have called the 'before times' – the time before the Covid pandemic. It was written in fits and starts before and through the pandemic itself. I am completing it as an unparalleled vaccination campaign against the virus is concluding in many, but sadly not all, parts of the world, and in the shadow of a catastrophic, savage and ferocious war on the European mainland.

These two events offer a dark mirror for some of the themes in this book. The war of conquest by Russia against Ukraine started as an attempt to annihilate Ukrainian national identity and to subsume Ukrainian territory within Russia itself. The direction of early wartime Russian propaganda, the inadvertent leaking of internal Russian security documents, widely circulated on social media, and statements by the Russian government generally pointed in a single direction: that Ukrainian national identity was to be dissolved within a greater Russian Federation. That is not what has happened. Ukrainian national identity instead seems to have been strengthened by the assault from without. The denial of a country's independent right to exist is a common trope, made with appeals to the force, strength and military might of the oppressor nation. Moreover, there are often outright denials that a country without an extended history has a right to exist. Statements can easily be found where it is alleged that one country has

a 'tenuous claim to nationhood',[1] but with the same author insist-
ing, without noticing any self-contradiction, that another nation
has a 'passionate attachment to their national identity. They fight
because they realise that, in defence of their freedom, their nation
is everything.'[2] Or where a professor of politics can tastelessly
declare, during the ongoing Russian war in Europe, that in future
'the British government would move to reclaim [by force of arms]
an island [Ireland] that some Tories believe belongs to Britain'.[3]
Are these simply foolish words, to be disowned or memory-holed
by their authors, similar to Orwell's *Nineteen Eighty-Four*, as their
foolishness becomes apparent to their authors? Or are they words
that some future demagogue will seek to build on?

Our memory of war and national adversity contrasts markedly
with our memory of pandemics or, indeed, other natural disasters.
It seems wars foster a national identity. Pandemics seem not to.
How will we *individually and collectively* remember and converse
together about our pandemic times? Will we imagine a post-
pandemic world? How will we imagine the next pandemic? How
will we understand the pandemics that didn't happen, because
governments took steps to ward them off before there was a problem in sight?

We humans are (somewhat) restless, novelty- and reward-
seeking, and hypersocial – with all of the usual outlets for these
drives denied us for long stretches during the lockdowns. Will we
remember a persistent sense of the ennui and dysphoria brought
on by the pandemic, mediated by chronic low-level stress and anxiety, exacerbated by social isolation and monotony? Or will we
treat it as a to-be-forgotten background hum?

We humans are not very good at remembering our past plagues,
but we are very good at remembering our past wars. We have con-
signed our plagues to history, and retain imperfect memories of
them – even across generations. My late grandfather was a victim
of polio, as was my wife's late great-aunt. They were infected
before Jonas Salk devised the first polio vaccine in the mid-1950s.

My grandfather wore a calliper on his leg all his life, and used a walking stick to get around; he never complained about it. Similarly uncomplaining, my wife's great-aunt spent months on end in hospital at a very young age, and she also needed special orthotic shoes and a walking stick. When asked, both would tolerantly recount their memories of those times – but only if asked.

The American historian Richard Melzer has noted a 'lapse of collective memory' surrounding the so-called Spanish Flu of the 1918–20 period, with few people remembering it, despite the vast death toll it exacted.[4] The cultural historian Elinor Accampo similarly says that while 'historians have given it [the Spanish Flu] ample attention . . . they have been at a loss to explain why such a cataclysmic event failed to register in public memory'.[5] Accampo further remarks that 'individuals experienced the flu privately rather than collectively' – it was hidden in ways that Covid is not in our hyperconnected age. Ida Milne, also a historian of the Spanish Flu, declares that 'Pandemics don't end with a bang – they end with a fizzle,' perhaps confounding our expectations for how this pandemic will end too.[6] I have deliberately said little in this book about the pandemic: there will, I hope, be a large literature to come on our collective and individual memories of these times. Our efforts to head off the next pandemic may, in part, be driven by our collective memories of the horrors of this one, and by our ability to engage in future mental time travel, where we imagine another preventable pandemic happening and work to prevent it.

ACKNOWLEDGEMENTS

My academic research concerns the brain systems supporting learning and memory, and how they are affected by stress and depression; to borrow a phrase, I am interested in understanding how 'the brain meets the world'. My previous books are best seen in that light too.

My ever-wise literary agent, Bill Hamilton of A. M. Heath, toiled through various discussions with me, and these resulted in a short proposal which found a receptive home with Stuart Williams of The Bodley Head, for which I am especially grateful.

There are many people to thank for discussions and for reading various drafts of this book: Bill Hamilton deserves my gratitude for his wise guidance, as do Stuart Williams and Connor Brown of The Bodley Head for careful readings and detailed feedback. Connor provided me with many detailed and incisive comments on the draft that helped me focus the text in, I hope, fruitful ways. Peter James also provided exacting and demanding readings, as well as important questions on specific points, all of which improved the text in so many ways, and for which I am particularly thankful.

I also want to thank especially Muireann Irish (The University of Sydney), Sean Commins (Maynooth University), Laurie Knell (Strategic Innovation Partners, and Trinity College Dublin), Vanesa Fischer (Trinity College Dublin), Vincent Walsh (University College,

London), and James Wertsch (Washington University, St Louis) for reading a draft, and for their very helpful suggestions and comments.

William (Bill) Lyons, Professor of Philosophy (Emeritus) at Trinity College Dublin, sent me a copy of his excellent book on introspection during the early phase of the pandemic lockdown, for which I am extremely grateful (note 1 of Chapter Two). I also thank Adrian Lynch (RTE) for some very useful and important conversations regarding Benedict Anderson while on night-time walks around coastal Dublin. I also want to mention Trinity College Dublin for being such a congenial place to work, with the intellectual freedom that attends a great university. Dalkey Library provided a congenial and quiet spot to work on many occasions, as did the Lexicon Library in Dun Laoghaire. Support your local libraries! They deserve it.

I also thank John Aggleton, FRS, of the University of Cardiff. We have worked together on the brain systems responsible for memory, supported by the Wellcome Trust, and I have drawn on a little of our thinking regarding our 'tripartite model of memory' in this book.

Susan Cantwell also provided fantastic secretarial support, which speeded the writing along.

NOTES

INTRODUCTION: WHAT HENRY TAUGHT US

1. Corkin, S. (2013). *Permanent Present Tense: The Man with No Memory, and What he Taught the World*. Allen Lane.

2. Papez, J. W. (1937). A proposed mechanism of emotion. *Archives of Neurology & Psychiatry*, 38(4), 725–43; but see Aggleton, J. P., Nelson, A. J. & O'Mara, S. M. (2022). Time to retire the serial Papez circuit: Implications for space, memory, and attention. *Neuroscience & Biobehavioral Reviews*, 104813.

3. Annese, J. et al. (2014). Postmortem examination of patient HM's brain based on histological sectioning and digital 3D reconstruction. *Nature Communications*, 5(1), 1–9, https://www.nature.com/articles/ncomms4122

4. Milner, B. (1970). Memory and the temporal regions of the brain. In K. H. Pribram & D. E. Broadbent (eds), *Biology of Memory*. New York: Academic Press.

5. Lawson, R. (1878). On the symptomatology of alcoholic brain disorders. *Brain*, 1(2), 182–94.

6. Lawson's contribution has been mostly overlooked by history, and has only been recently redescribed: Kopelman, M. D. (1995). The Korsakoff Syndrome. *British Journal of Psychiatry*, 166, 154–73; Aggleton, J. P. & O'Mara, S. M. (2022). The anterior thalamic nuclei: core components of a tripartite episodic memory system. *Nature Reviews Neuroscience*, 1–12, https://www.nature.com/articles/s41583-022-00591-8

7. Korsakoff, S. S. (1887). Ob alkogol'nom paraliche (Of alcoholic paralysis: disturbance of psychic activity and its relation to the disturbance of the psychic sphere in multiple neuritis of nonalcoholic origin). *Vestnik Klin. Psychiat. Neurol.*, 4, 1–102.

8. Aggleton & O'Mara (2022), The anterior thalamic nuclei.

9. Kopelman, M. D. (1987). Two types of confabulation. *Journal of Neurology, Neurosurgery & Psychiatry*, 50(11), 1482–7; Schnider, A. (2003). Spontaneous confabulation and the adaptation of thought to ongoing reality. *Nature Reviews Neuroscience*, 4(8), 662–71.

10. Dalla Barba, G., Cipolotti, L. & Denes, G. (1990). Autobiographical memory loss and confabulation in Korsakoff's syndrome: a case report. *Cortex*, 26(4), 525–34.

11. Borsutzky, S., Fujiwara, E., Brand, M. & Markowitsch, H. J. (2008). Confabulations in alcoholic Korsakoff patients. *Neuropsychologia*, 46(13), 3133–43.

12. The confabulation phase often resolves in such patients, and when it doesn't they often have additional damage to other brain regions: Kopelman, M. D. et al. (2009). The Korsakoff Syndrome: Clinical Aspects, Psychology and Treatment. *Alcohol and Alcoholism*, 44, 148–54, https://doi.org/10.1093/alcalc/agn118

13. Rajaram, S. and Pereira-Pasarin, L. P. (2010). Collaborative Memory: Cognitive Research and Theory. *Perspect. Psychol. Sci.*, 5(6), 649–63, https://doi.org/10.1177/1745691610388763, PMID: 26161882

14. Corkin (2013), *Permanent Present Tense*.

15. Harris, P. L. (2012). *Trusting What You're Told: How Children Learn from Others*. Cambridge, Mass.: Harvard University Press.

16. Brashier, N. M. & Marsh, E. J. (2020). Judging truth. *Annu. Rev. Psychol.*, 71, 499–515.

17. Harry G. Frankfurt (2005). *On Bullshit*. Princeton University Press.

18. Higgins, E. T., Rossignac-Milon, M. & Echterhoff, G. (2021). Shared Reality: From Sharing-Is-Believing to Merging Minds. *Current Directions in Psychological Science*, 30(2), 103–10, https://doi.org/10.1177/0963721421992027

19. Ibid.

20. Ibid., p. 103.

21. There is an interesting and accessible literature on the psychology of those who espouse conspiracy theories: e.g. Douglas, K. M., Sutton, R. M. & Cichocka, A. (2017). The psychology of conspiracy theories. *Current Directions in Psychological Science*, 26(6), 538–42; De Coninck, D. et al. (2021). Beliefs in conspiracy theories and misinformation about COVID-19: Comparative perspectives on the role of anxiety, depression and exposure to and trust in information sources. *Frontiers in Psychology*, 12, 646394; https://ec.europa.eu/info/live-work-travel-eu/coronavirus-response/fighting-disinformation/identifying-conspiracy-theories_en; van Prooijen, J. W. and Douglas, K. M. (2018), Belief in conspiracy theories: Basic principles of an emerging research domain. *Eur. J. Soc. Psychol.*, 48(7), 897–908, https://doi.org/10.1002/ejsp.2530

22. Here's a handy dynamic listing: https://en.wikipedia.org/wiki/List_of_conspiracy_theories

23. Uscinski, J., Enders, A., Klofstad, C., Seelig, M., Drochon, H. et al. (2022). Have beliefs in conspiracy theories increased over time? *PLOS ONE*, 17(7), e0270429, https://doi.org/10.1371/journal.pone.0270429

24. Hirst, W., & Coman, A. (2018). Building a collective memory: The case for collective forgetting. *Current Opinion in Psychology*, 23, 88–92.

25. Atran, Scott (2022). The will to fight: Throughout history, the most effective combatants have powered to victory on commitment to core values and collective resolve, https://aeon.co/essays/wars-are-won-by-people-willing-to-fight-for-comrade-and-cause

26. Raichle, M. E. et al. (2001). A default mode of brain function. *Proceedings of the National Academy of Sciences*, 98(2), 676–82; Poerio, G. L. et al. (2017). The role of the default mode network in component processes underlying the wandering mind. *Social Cognitive and Affective Neuroscience*, 12, 1047–62, https://doi.org/10.1093/scan/nsx041

27. https://www.nytimes.com/2015/11/01/opinion/sunday/the-light-beam-rider.html#:~:text=While%20there%2C%20Einstein%20tried%20to,the%20wave%20would%20seem%20stationary; https://www.nationalgeographic.com/science/article/einstein-relativity-thought-experiment-train-lightning-genius

28. The quote as it stands is intoned by 'Hans Gruber' (Alan Rickman) in the movie *Die Hard* (1988), and is a mash-up of several different quotes from differing eras: https://www.theparisreview.org/blog/2020/03/19/and-alexander-wept/

1: HAVING CONVERSATIONS WITH OTHERS

1. Levinson, S. C. & Torreira, F. (2015). Timing in turn-taking and its implications for processing models of language. *Frontiers in Psychology*, 6, 731, https://www.frontiersin.org/articles/10.3389/fpsyg.2015.00731/full

2. Donnelly, S. & Kidd, E. (2021). The Longitudinal Relationship between Conversational Turn-Taking and Vocabulary Growth in Early Language Development. *Child Development*, 92, 609–25; Bateson, M. C. (1975). Mother–infant exchanges: The epigenesis of conversational interaction. *Annals of the New York Academy of Sciences*, 263, 101–13, https://doi.org/10.1111/j.1749-6632.1975.tb41575.x

3. De Vos, C. (2018). Rapid turn-taking as a constant feature of signed conversations, http://evolang.org/torun/proceedings/paperpdfs/Evolang_12_paper_107.pdf

4. Mehl, M. R. et al. (2007). Are women really more talkative than men? *Science*, 317(5834), 82.

5. Heldner, M. & Edlund, J. (2010). Pauses, gaps and overlaps in conversations. *Journal of Phonetics*, 38(4), 555–68; Bögels, S. & Levinson, S. C. (2017). The brain behind the response: Insights into turn-taking in conversation from neuroimaging. *Research on Language and Social Interaction*, 50(1), 71–89.

6. Harland, M. J. & Steele, J. R. (1997). Biomechanics of the sprint start. *Sports Medicine*, 23(1), 11–20; Mirshams Shahshahani, P. et al. (2018). On the apparent decrease in Olympic sprinter reaction times. *PLOS ONE*, 13(6), e0198633.

7. Levinson, S. C. (2016). Turn-taking in human communication – origins and implications for language processing. *Trends in Cognitive Sciences*, 20(1), 6–14.

8. Conversations are, of course, highly flexible, because multiple speakers can participate. Here I'm keeping it to a conversational dyad – i.e. two people – for ease of description.

9. Levinson, S. C. & Holler, J. (2014). The origin of human multi-modal communication. *Philosophical Transactions of the Royal Society B: Biological Sciences*, 369(1651), 20130302.

10. Dediu, D. et al. (2021). The vocal tract as a time machine: inferences about past speech and language from the anatomy of the speech organs. *Philosophical Transactions of the Royal Society B: Biological Sciences*, 376(1824), 20200192.

11: Chow, C. P. et al. (2015). Vocal turn-taking in a non-human primate is learned during ontogeny. *Proceedings of the Royal Society B: Biological Sciences*, 282(1807), 20150069.

12. Bögels, S. et al. (2015). Neural signatures of response planning occur midway through an incoming question in conversation. *Scientific Reports*, 5, 12881.

13. This rating process is needed so that the EEG can be analysed and timed from the uttering of that particular word for each question asked, and the electrical signal from the brain tested at that word for significant changes in the electrical signal of the brain.

14. Nora, A. et al. (2020). Dynamic time-locking mechanism in the cortical representation of spoken words. *eNeuro*, 7(4), https://www.eneuro.org/content/7/4/ENEURO.0475-19.2020

15. Wang, Y. C. et al. (2021). Predictive Neural Computations Support Spoken Word Recognition: Evidence from MEG and Competitor Priming. *Journal of Neuroscience*, 41(32), 6919–32. This study uses Bayes' rule – a way of combining information about a particular event with prior knowledge to make predictions about that event.

16. Yeager, D. S. & Krosnick, J. A. (2011). Does mentioning 'some people' and 'other people' in a survey question increase the accuracy of adolescents' self-reports? *Developmental Psychology*, 47(6), 1674.

17. Huang, F. L. & Cornell, D. G. (2015). The impact of definition and question order on the prevalence of bullying victimization using student self-reports. *Psychological Assessment*, 27(4), 1484; they used a sample of 17,301 students attending 119 high schools in the USA, with participants randomised according to question type.

18. Broockman, D. & Kalla, J. (2016). Durably reducing transphobia: A field experiment on door-to-door canvassing. *Science*, 352(6282), 220–4; Kalla, J. L., Levine, A. S. & Broockman, D. (2021). Personalizing moral reframing in interpersonal conversation: A field experiment. *Journal of Politics*, https://www.journals.uchicago.edu/doi/abs/10.1086/716944?journalCode=jop. See also: Resnick, Brian (2020). How to talk someone out of bigotry, https://www.vox.com/2020/1/29/21065620/broockman-kalla-deep-canvassing and https://deepcanvass.org/

19. O'Mara, S. (2022). Political memories (no punditry; just memory and identity), https://brainpizza.substack.com/p/political-memories

20. Yeomans, M. et al. (2020). Conversational receptiveness: Improving engagement with opposing views. *Organizational Behavior and Human Decision Processes*, 160, 131–48.

21. Gabbert, F. et al. (2021). Exploring the use of rapport in professional information-gathering contexts by systematically mapping the evidence base. *Applied Cognitive Psychology*, 35(2), 329–41.

22. Meissner, C. A. et al. (2017). Developing an evidence-based perspective on inter-rogation: A review of the US government's high-value detainee interrogation group research program. *Psychology, Public Policy, and Law*, 23(4), 438; O'Mara, S. (2019). Interrogating the brain: Torture and the neuroscience of humane interrogation. In Steven J. Barela, Mark Fallon, Gloria Gaggioli & Jens David Ohlin (eds), *Interrogation and Torture: Research on Efficacy and its Integration with Morality and Legality*. New York: Oxford University Press.

23. Worsfold, Chris (2019). 'On opening the clinical encounter', https://www.chris worsfold.com/on-opening-the-clinical-encounter/

24. This discussion draws especially on the pioneering and important work of William Hirst and Gerald Echterhoff (2012), Remembering in conversations: The social shar-ing and reshaping of memories. *Ann. Rev. Psych.*, 63, 55–79, https://www.annual reviews.org/doi/full/10.1146/annurev-psych-120710-100340

25. https://quoteinvestigator.com/2011/08/26/reinforcements/

26. Hirst and Echterhoff (2012), Remembering in conversations.

27. Pasupathi, M. et al. (2009). To tell or not to tell: Disclosure and the narrative self. *Journal of Personality*, 77(1), 89–124.

28. Harber, K. D. & Cohen, D. J. (2005). The emotional broadcaster theory of social sharing. *Journal of Language and Social Psychology*, 24(4), 382–400.

29. Skagerberg, E. M. & Wright, D. B. (2008). The prevalence of co-witnesses and co-witness discussions in real eyewitnesses. *Psychology, Crime & Law*, 14(6), 513–21.

30. Hirst and Echterhoff summarise this view as follows: we humans engage in a 'constant chatter [which] can be about jointly experienced events, individually experi-enced events, or facts': Hirst and Echterhoff (2012), Remembering in conversations.

31. Collins, A. (2006). The embodiment of reconciliation: Order and change in the work of Frederic Bartlett. *History of Psychology*, 9(4), 290; Bartlett, F. C. (1916). An experimental study of some problems of perceiving and imagining. *British Journal of Psychology*, 8, 222–66.

32. Generally, Americans use the term 'liberal' to refer to progressive policies and social equality, while Europeans uses the term to refer to free-market economics and limited government intervention.

33. Hirst and Echterhoff (2012), Remembering in conversations, p. 71

34. Genetic lineages are not necessarily your friend, as they may uncover diverse and unexpected genetic influences on your own personal genome!

35. And to annoy the racists, all human lineages are ultimately out of Africa.

36. Tulving, E. (1985). Memory and Consciousness. *Canadian Psychology* 26, 1–12, https://www.apa.org/pubs/journals/features/cap-h0080017.pdf; here's a nice intro-duction to Tulving's thought: https://www.apa.org/monitor/oct03/mental; see also Suddendorf, T. & Corballis, M. C. (1997). Mental time travel and the evolution of the human mind. *Genetic, Social, and General Psychology Monographs*, 123, 133–67;

Suddendorf, T. et al. (2009). Mental time travel and the shaping of the human mind. *Philosophical Transactions of the Royal Society B: Biological Sciences*, 364(1521), 1317–24, https://www.ncbi.nlm.nih.gov/pmc/articles/PMC2666704/

37. A biblical reference (Exodus 3:8); it was invoked by a Brexiter Tory MP regarding the economic prospects of the UK after its departure from the EU (https://www.joe.ie/news/watch-british-mp-thought-entitled-irish-passport-back-nonsense-645640).

38. Hirst and Echterhoff (2012), Remembering in conversations.

39. Squire, L. R. (2009). The legacy of patient H.M. for neuroscience. *Neuron*, 61, 6–9, https://www.ncbi.nlm.nih.gov/pmc/articles/PMC2649674/; Wikipedia does a very readable introduction here: https://en.wikipedia.org/wiki/Henry_Molaison

2: THE BUZZ OF MENTAL LIFE: THE CONVERSATIONS WITHIN US

1. Lyons, William E. (1986). *The Disappearance of Introspection*. Cambridge, Mass.: MIT Press/Bradford Books.

2. Asthana, Hari Shanker (2015). 'Wilhelm Wundt'. *Psychological Studies*, 60, 244–8, https://doi.org/10.1007/s12646-014-0295-1

3. I must confess to not particularly enjoying Henry James's writing – unlike his brother William, who is very readable (albeit in small doses). The last James novel I read was *The Portrait of a Lady*, which left me feeling that had it been half the length, it would have been twice as good.

4. This is at best an approximation: the reality is reflected in the following paper's title: Poeppel, D. & Idsardi, W. (2022). We don't know how the brain stores anything, let alone words. *Trends in Cognitive Sciences*, https://www.sciencedirect.com/science/article/pii/S1364661322002066

5. Ramsey, N. F. et al. (2018). Decoding spoken phonemes from sensorimotor cortex with high-density ECoG grids. *Neuroimage*, 180, 301–11; Staresina, B. P. & Wimber, M. (2019). A neural chronometry of memory recall. *Trends in Cognitive Sciences*, 23(12), 1071–85, https://www.sciencedirect.com/science/article/pii/S1364661319302359

6. Baumeister, R. F. et al. (2020). Everyday thoughts in time: Experience sampling studies of mental time travel. *Personality and Social Psychology Bulletin*, 46(12), 1631–48, https://journals.sagepub.com/doi/pdf/10.1177/0146167220908411

7. Kahneman, D. (2011). *Thinking, Fast and Slow*. Macmillan, https://www.ted.com/talks/daniel_kahneman_the_riddle_of_experience_vs_memory/

8. Burkeman, O. (2012). *The Antidote: Happiness for People Who Can't Stand Positive Thinking*. Bodley Head. I'm not certain he's correct, as the following study seems to show: Prati, A. & Senik, C. (2022). Feeling Good Is Feeling Better. *Psychological Science*, 33(11), 1828–41, https://doi.org/10.1177/09567976221096158. Prati and Senik analysed data from four countries over a period of several decades, finding that people tend to overestimate how much happier they are now compared to the past, *and underestimate how happy they were in the past*. However, happy people remember the past as being worse than it was, and unhappy people remember it as better. Burkeman's intuition may depend on who you ask!

9. Baird, B., Smallwood, J., Mrazek, M. D., Kam, J. W., Franklin, M. S. & Schooler, J. W. (2012). Inspired by distraction: Mind wandering facilitates creative incubation. *Psychological Science*, 23(10), 1117–22.

10. Wang, H. T. et al. (2018). Dimensions of experience: exploring the heterogeneity of the wandering mind. *Psychological Science*, 29(1), 56–71, https://journals.sagepub.com/doi/full/10.1177/0956797617728727

11. Baumeister et al. (2020), Everyday thoughts in time.

12. Speer, M. E. et al. (2014). Savoring the past: positive memories evoke value representations in the striatum. *Neuron*, 84(4), 847–56; Oba, K. et al. (2016). Memory and reward systems coproduce 'nostalgic' experiences in the brain. *Social, Cognitive, and Affective Neuroscience*, 11(7), 1069–77.

13. Speer, M. E. & Delgado, M. R. (2017). Reminiscing about positive memories buffers acute stress responses. *Nature Human Behaviour*, 1(5), 1–9, https://www.ncbi.nlm.nih.gov/pmc/articles/PMC6719713/

14. Köber, C. & Habermas, T. (2017). How stable is the personal past? Stability of most important autobiographical memories and life narratives across eight years in a life span sample. *Journal of Personality and Social Psychology*, 113, 608–26, http://doi.org/10.1037/pspp0000145; they originally recruited their participants for testing in 2003; they were then tested again in 2007 and 2011. They examined a group of 164 adults of six differing age groups in three waves, over an eight-year period. The age cohorts tested were at ages eight, twelve, sixteen and twenty.

15. D'Argembeau, A. (2016). The role of personal goals in future-oriented mental time travel. In K. Michaelian, S. B. Klein & K. K. Szpunar (eds), *Seeing the Future: Theoretical Perspectives on Future-Oriented Mental Time Travel*. Oxford University Press, 199–214, https://doi.org/10.1093/acprof:oso/9780190241537.003.0010; D'Argembeau, A. (2018). Mind-Wandering and Self-referential Thought. In Kieran C. R. Fox and Kalina Christoff (eds), *The Oxford Handbook of Spontaneous Thought: Mind-Wandering, Creativity, and Dreaming*. Oxford University Press, 181–91, https://orbi.uliege.be/handle/2268/209353

16. McCormick, C. et al. (2018). Mind-wandering in people with hippocampal damage. *Journal of Neuroscience*, 38, 2745–54, https://www.jneurosci.org/content/38/11/2745?etoc=

17. Intriguingly, people who have the condition known as 'aphantasia', where they seemingly lack visual imagery, also seem to have at least some deficits in mental time travel, and report less rich autobiographical memory: Dawes, A. J. et al. (2020). A cognitive profile of multi-sensory imagery, memory and dreaming in aphantasia. *Scientific Reports*, 10, 1–10, https://www.nature.com/articles/s41598-020-65705-7

18. They conducted twenty such probes for each patient over two eight-hour days, at the same times, in the same rooms, etc. The shadowing research assistant would ask participants what was on their minds just prior to their being asked, and their responses were recorded on response sheets (they were given one minute to speak about what was on their minds). The samples were then all coded in terms of the type and content of thoughts the patients (and controls) were having in the moments prior to the probe.

3: SOLVING PROBLEMS TOGETHER: BEES DO IT, THE BORG DO IT AND WE DO IT TOO

1. 'Induced demand' is a thing, though: the build 'one more lane to fix it' meme is on point – https://mobile.twitter.com/urbanthoughts11/status/1569068607014932481 – because building ever more roads creates ever more traffic and exurban sprawl. The answer is structural – building great public transport for everyone, and making it cheap to use.

2. Willer, R. (2009). Groups reward individual sacrifice: The status solution to the collective action problem. *American Sociological Review*, 74, 23–43; Ostrom, Elinor (1990). *Governing the Commons: The Evolution of Institutions for Collective Action*. New York: Cambridge University Press.

3. Vlasceanu, M. et al. (2018). Cognition in a social context: a social-interactionist approach to emergent phenomena. *Current Directions in Psychological Science*, 27(5), 369–77.

4. Vlasceanu, M. et al. (2021). Network Structure Impacts the Synchronization of Collective Beliefs. *Journal of Cognition and Culture*, 21, 431–48, https://doi.org/10.1163/15685373-12340120

5. https://en.wikipedia.org/wiki/Transport_in_Greater_Tokyo#:~:text=40%20million%20passengers%20(counted%20twice,8.66%20million%20using%20it%20daily

6. Johnson, B. R. & Linksvayer, T. A. (2010). Deconstructing the superorganism: social physiology, ground plans, and sociogenomics. *Quarterly Review of Biology*, 85, 57–79, https://www.jstor.org/stable/pdf/10.1086/650290.pdf

7. Coronavirus: Outcry after Trump suggests injecting disinfectant as treatment, https://www.bbc.com/news/world-us-canada-52407177

8. Paton Walsh, N., Shelley, J., Duwe, E. and Bonnett, W. (2020). Bolsonaro calls coronavirus a 'little flu'. Inside Brazil's hospitals, doctors know the horrifying reality. CNN, Updated 0656 GMT (1456 HKT), 25 May, https://edition.cnn.com/2020/05/23/americas/brazil-coronavirus-hospitals-intl/index.html

9. This study estimates twice as fatal: Ludwig, M. et al. (2021). Clinical outcomes and characteristics of patients hospitalized for Influenza or COVID-19 in Germany. *International Journal of Infectious Diseases*, 103, 316–22, https://www.sciencedirect.com/science/article/pii/S1201971220325200; van Asten, L. et al. (2021) suggest a fatality rate in the initial wave of 1%: Excess Deaths during Influenza and Coronavirus Disease and Infection-Fatality Rate for Severe Acute Respiratory Syndrome Coronavirus 2, the Netherlands. *Emerg. Infect. Dis.*, 27(2), 411–20, https://doi.

org/10.3201/eid2702.202999, ePub 2021 Jan 4, https://www.ncbi.nlm.nih.gov/pmc/articles/PMC7853586/. How many people does that 1% translate to on your street? They also say deaths were 'mitigated by nonpharmaceutical control measures' (i.e. masks and social distancing). If you think otherwise, publish your mathematical and statistical model, data and code in a peer-reviewed journal, please, for all to see. And adhere to best-practice open-science policies on data transparency. See also: COVID-19 is a leading cause of death in children and young people in the US, https://www.ox.ac.uk/news/2023-01-31-covid-19-leading-cause-death-children-and-young-people-us. No doubt the debate will continue, until people get bored and move on to something else, leaving this for the medical statisticians and medical historians.

10. Rabb, N. et al. (2019). Individual Representation in a Community of Knowledge. *Trends in Cognitive Sciences*, 23, 891–902, https://www.sciencedirect.com/science/article/pii/S1364661319301998

11. This remark was originally made by a UK politician, Michael Gove, who was apparently unhappy that expert economists did not back Brexit. He was quoted as saying 'people in this country have had enough of experts' (Mance, H. (2016). 'Britain has had enough of experts, says Gove'. *Financial Times*, 3 June, https://www.ft.com/content/3be49734-29cb-11e6-83e4-abc22d5d108c). The expert economists do appear to have been correct: https://edition.cnn.com/2022/12/24/economy/brexit-uk-economy/index.html#:~:text=Permanent%20damage%20to%20trade&text=By%20contrast%2C%20the%20UK%20Office,lower%20in%20the%20long%20run. See also Hawkins, Amy (2016). Has the public really had enough of experts? https://fullfact.org/blog/2016/sep/has-public-really-had-enough-experts/

12. Rabb et al. (2019), Individual Representation in a Community of Knowledge.

13. Excess Death Rates for Republicans and Democrats during the COVID-19 Pandemic, https://www.nber.org/papers/w30512; https://mobile.twitter.com/paulgp/status/1576899935147991041

14. https://www.psychologicalscience.org/news/repeating-misinformation-doesnt-make-it-true-but-does-make-it-more-likely-to-be-believed.html; https://www.apa.org/monitor/2017/05/alternative-facts; https://www.bbc.com/future/article/20161026-how-liars-create-the-illusion-of-truth; Fazio, L. K. et al. (2015). Knowledge does not protect against illusory truth. *Journal of Experimental Psychology: General*, 144, 993.

15. Simons, D. J. and C. F. Chabris (2011). What People Believe about How Memory Works: A Representative Survey of the U.S. Population. *PLOS ONE*, 6(8), e22757, https://doi.org/10.1371/journal.pone.0022757

16. Hassan, A. & Barber, S. J. (2021). The effects of repetition frequency on the illusory truth effect. *Cognitive Research: Principles and Implications*, 6, 1–12, https://cognitiveresearchjournal.springeropen.com/articles/10.1186/s41235-021-00301-5; see also https://thedecisionlab.com/biases/illusory-truth-effect/. I have found people can often become quite aggrieved when they say these kinds of things, and then ask me, as a neuroscientist, to confirm what they say is true, and I can't and won't – for they are empirically unmoored assertions, owing lots to fancy and little to fact.

17. Paton Walsh et al. (2020). Bolsonaro calls coronavirus a 'little flu'. Inside Brazil's hospitals, doctors know the horrifying reality.

18. Rabb et al. (2019), Individual Representation in a Community of Knowledge.

19. https://www.azquotes.com/quote/1258713

20. Ibid.

21. https://powerofus.substack.com/p/beyond-tribalism

22. Although https://www.buzzfeednews.com/article/otilliasteadman/mad-mike-hughes-rocket-death-flat-earth

23. Sins of Memory: false memory implantation in adults is easy (bonus: here's one way to do it), https://brainpizza.substack.com/p/sins-of-memory

24. Edelson, M. et al. (2011). Following the Crowd: Brain Substrates of Long-Term Memory Conformity. *Science*, 333(6038), 108–11, http://www.weizmann.ac.il/neuro biology/labs/dudai/uploads/files/Science-2011-Edelson-108-11.pdf

25. Dunbar, R. I. (2004). Gossip in evolutionary perspective. *Review of General Psychology*, 8(2), 100–10, https://journals.sagepub.com/doi/full/10.1037/1089-2680.8.2.100

26. Babaei Aghbolagh, M. & Sattari Ardabili, F. (2016). An overview of the social functions of gossip in the hospitals. Available at SSRN 3347590, https://papers.ssrn.com/sol3/papers.cfm?abstract_id=3347590

27. McAndrew, F. T. (2016). Gossip is a social skill – not a character flaw, https://theconversation.com/gossip-is-a-social-skill-not-a-character-flaw-51629

28. Feinberg, M. et al. (2012). The virtues of gossip: reputational information sharing as prosocial behavior. *Journal of Personality and Social Psychology*, 102, 1015–30, https://doi.org/10.1037/a0026650; Feinberg, M. et al. (2014). Gossip and Ostracism Promote Cooperation in Groups. *Psychological Science*, 25(3), 656–64, https://doi.org/10.1177/0956797613510184

29. Demerath, L. & Korotayev, A. V. (2015). The importance of gossip across societies: correlations with institutionalization. *Cross-Cultural Research*, 49(3), 297–314.

4: CONSTRUCTING SHARED COGNITIVE REALITIES TOGETHER: NONSENSE SYLLABLES AND WARRING GHOSTS

1. https://psychclassics.yorku.ca/Ebbinghaus/index.htm

2. Fraisse, P. (1957). *Psychologie du temps*. Paris: PUF (http://www.nuorisotutkimus seura.fi/images/julkaisuja/rype2/3/2.html).

3. Now styled the MRC Cognition and Brain Sciences Unit: https://www.mrc-cbu.cam.ac.uk/

4. Bartlett, F. C. (1932). *Remembering: A Study in Experimental and Social Psychology*. Cambridge University Press.

5. Bartlett adapted this story from an original collected and translated in 1891 by the German-American anthropologist Franz Boas. Bartlett's account is at Bartlett, F. C.

(1920). Some experiments on the reproduction of folk-stories. *Folklore*, 31(1), 30–47; the Boas translation is at Boas, Franz (1901). *Bureau of American Ethnology*, Bulletin 26, 182–4, https://archive.org/details/bulletin261901smit/page/182/mode/2up? view=theater

6. Ibid.

7. Some questions were misleading: there was no mention of a boat, or a bow, and the warriors were going upriver, not downriver.

8. Halbwachs, M. (1992). *On Collective Memory*. University of Chicago Press, p. 42

9. Ibid., p. 51.

10. Schudson, M. (1995). Dynamics of distortion in collective memory. In D. L. Schacter & J. T. Coyle (eds) (1997), *Memory Distortion: How Minds, Brains, and Societies Reconstruct the Past*. Cambridge, Mass.: Harvard University Press.

11. Olick, J. K. (1999). Collective memory: the two cultures. *Sociological Theory*, 7, 333–48, https://journals.sagepub.com/doi/pdf/10.1111/0735-2751.00083

12. Aggleton & O'Mara (2022), The anterior thalamic nuclei.

13. Hoel, Erik (2021). How to make art that lasts 1,000 years: On creating for the Long Now, https://erikhoel.substack.com/p/how-to-make-art-that-lasts-1000-years

14. Roediger III, H. L. & Abel, M. (2015). Collective memory: A new arena of cognitive study. *Trends in Cognitive Sciences*, 19, 359–61.

15. At least within a US test sample. Roediger, H. L. & DeSoto, K. A. (2014). Forgetting the presidents. *Science*, 346(6213), 1106–9.

16. The effect is named for the German psychiatrist Hedwig von Restorff, who first described the effect in her 1933 paper Über die Wirkung von Bereichsbildungen im Spurenfeld [The effects of field formation in the trace field]. *Psychologische Forschung* [Psychological Research] (in German), 18(1), 299–342. Wiki carries a short biography, emphasising the importance of the effect at https://en.wikipedia.org/wiki/Hedwig_ von_Restorff

17. Lee, H., Bellana, B. & Chen, J. (2020). What can narratives tell us about the neural bases of human memory? *Current Opinion in Behavioral Sciences*, 32, 111–19; US Bureau of Labor Statistics: American Time Use Survey (2018), https://www.bls.gov/news. release/pdf/atus.pdf

18. Smith, D. et al. (2017). Cooperation and the evolution of hunter-gatherer storytelling. *Nature Communications*, 8, 1–9, https://www.nature.com/articles/s41467-017-02036-8

19. See http://jchenlab.johnshopkins.edu/ and https://scholar.google.com/citations? user=mOwF8UEAAAAJ&hl=en&oi=sra

20. In this way it is possible to think of movies as a 'stimulus class' for brain imaging.

21. Zadbood, A. et al. (2017). How we transmit memories to other brains: constructing shared neural representations via communication. *Cerebral Cortex*, 27(10), 4988–5000.

22. Lee, H. et al. (2020). What can narratives tell us about the neural bases of human memory? *Current Opinion in Behavioral Sciences*, 32, 111–19.

23. I make this case at length in O'Mara, S. (2019). *In Praise of Walking: The New Science of How We Walk and Why It's Good for Us*. London/New York: Bodley Head.
24. Aggleton and O'Mara (2022), The anterior thalamic nuclei.

5: CONVERSATIONS ABOUT POSSIBLE
PASTS AND ALTERNATIVE FUTURES

1. Wagenaar, W. A. (1986). My memory: A study of autobiographical memory over six years. *Cognitive Psychology*, 18(2), 225–52. See also Sotgiu, I. (2021). Eight memory researchers investigating their own autobiographical memory. *Applied Cognitive Psychology*, 35, 1631–40 for an account of seven other memory researchers (Francis Galton, Madorah Smith, Marigold Linton, Steen Larsen, Dorthe Berntsen, Alan Baddeley and Richard White) who undertook variations and precursor investigations of their own autobiographical memories (available at https://onlinelibrary.wiley.com/doi/full/10.1002/acp.3888).

2. Wagenaar (1986), My memory, p. 229

3. Weil, S. (1997). *Gravity and Grace*. Lincoln, Nebr.: University of Nebraska Press, p. 105.

4. Quoidbach, J. et al. (2013). The end of history illusion. *Science*, 339(6115), 96–8, https://science.sciencemag.org/content/sci/339/6115/96.full.pdf

5. Kahneman (2011), *Thinking, Fast and Slow*.

6. Muireann was my PhD student at the Trinity College Institute of Neuroscience; she is now Professor of Cognitive Neuroscience at the University of Sydney: https://www.sydney.edu.au/science/about/our-people/academic-staff/muireann-irish.html

7. Irish, M. & Piguet, O. (2013). The pivotal role of semantic memory in remembering the past and imagining the future. *Frontiers in Behavioral Neuroscience*, 7, 27, https://www.frontiersin.org/articles/10.3389/fnbeh.2013.00027/full; Irish, M. et al. (2011). Impaired capacity for autonoetic reliving during autobiographical event recall in mild Alzheimer's disease. *Cortex*, 47(2), 236–49.

8. See also Irish, M. et al. (2012). Considering the role of semantic memory in episodic future thinking: evidence from semantic dementia. *Brain*, 135(7), 2178–91, https://doi.org/10.1093/brain/aws119, ePub 2012 May 21, PMID: 22614246.

9. Lima, B. S. et al. (2020). Impaired coherence for semantic but not episodic autobiographical memory in semantic variant primary progressive aphasia. *Cortex*, 123, 72–85. This type of study requires selecting the appropriate patients, based on clinical and other criteria, into the correct group and then probing their autobiographical memories and their semantic memories. This can be done using a standardised clinical interview known as the 'autobiographical interview', which can be supplemented by recording and then analysing the speech of these differing groups, and comparing speech patterns in these groups relative to appropriately matched controls.

10. Brinthaupt, T. M. & Dove, C. T. (2012). Differences in self-talk frequency as a function of age, only-child, and imaginary childhood companion status. *Journal of Research in Personality*, 46, 326–33.

11. Nelson, K. & Fivush, R. (2004). The emergence of autobiographical memory: a social cultural developmental theory. *Psychological Review*, 111, 486.

12. Wu, Y. & Jobson, L. (2019). Maternal reminiscing and child autobiographical memory elaboration: A meta-analytic review. *Dev. Psychol.*, 55, 2505–21.

6: HOW CONVERSATION SHAPES SHARED REALITIES

1. Hirst and Echterhoff (2012), Remembering in conversations.

2. Wegner, D. M. et al. (1991). Transactive memory in close relationships. *Journal of Personality and Social Psychology*, 61(6), 923, http://citeseerx.ist.psu.edu/viewdoc/download?doi=10.1.1.466.8153&rep=rep1&type=pdf

3. Barnier, A. J. et al. (2018). Collaborative facilitation in older couples: Successful joint remembering across memory tasks. *Frontiers in Psychology*, 9, 2385.

4. Horschler, D. J., MacLean, E. L. & Santos, L. R. (2020). Do non-human primates really represent others' beliefs? *Trends in Cognitive Sciences*, 24(8), 594–605, https://www.sciencedirect.com/science/article/abs/pii/S1364661320301339

5. Meade, M. L. et al. (2009). Expertise promotes facilitation on a collaborative memory task. *Memory*, 17, 39–48.

6. https://en.wikipedia.org/wiki/MMR_vaccine_and_autism – this offers an excellent account of the controversy.

7. https://www.hse.ie/eng/health/immunisation/pubinfo/pcischedule/vpds/mmr/: for example, 'If 1000 people get measles, 1 or 2 will die; 1 will develop encephalitis (swelling of the brain); for every 10 children who develop encephalitis, 1 will die and up to 4 will have brain damage' (much more at this link); see also https://www.cdc.gov/vaccinesafety/vaccines/mmr-vaccine.html

8. Quick, V. B. S. et al. (2021). Leveraging large genomic datasets to illuminate the pathobiology of autism spectrum disorders. *Neuropsychopharmacology*, 46, 55–69; Khundrakpam, B. et al. (2020). Neural correlates of polygenic risk score for autism spectrum disorders in general population. *Brain Communications*, 2(2), fcaa092; Veatch, O. J. et al. (2014). Genetically meaningful phenotypic subgroups in autism spectrum disorders. *Genes, Brain and Behavior*, 13(3), 276–85; Willsey, A. J. & State, M. W. (2015). Autism spectrum disorders: from genes to neurobiology. *Current Opinion in Neurobiology*, 30, 92–9; Fu, Jack M. et al. (2021). Rare coding variation illuminates the allelic architecture, risk genes, cellular expression patterns, and phenotypic context of autism, https://www.medrxiv.org/content/10.1101/2021.12.20.21267194v1

9. For example: https://www.cochranelibrary.com/cdsr/doi/10.1002/14651858.CD004407.pub4/full

10. For Tolstoy's *What is Art?* see https://www.penguin.co.uk/books/35255/what-is-art-/9780140446425.html

11. https://www.psychologytoday.com/ie/blog/living-single/201411/telling-lies-fact-fiction-and-nonsense-maria-hartwig; Vrij, A., Hartwig, M. & Granhag, P. A. (2019). Reading Lies: Nonverbal Communication and Deception. *Annu. Rev. Psychol.*, 70, 295–317, https://doi.org/10.1146/annurev-psych-010418-103135, PMID: 30609913

12. Edelson, M. et al. (2011). Following the crowd: brain substrates of long-term memory conformity. *Science*, 333(6038), 108–11.

13. Studies involving deception or misdirection of human participants have long been the subject of ethical debate, and they arise in many domains. In clinical medicine, for example, you may not know if you are assigned to an 'active ingredient' or placebo group in a studies of drug action or of vaccine efficacy. For discussions see, for example, Boynton, M. H. et al. (2013). Exploring the ethics and psychological impact of deception in psychological research. *IRB*, 35(2), 7–13, https://www.ncbi.nlm.nih.gov/pmc/articles/PMC4502434/; Miller, F. G. & Kaptchuk, T. J. (2008). Deception of subjects in neuroscience: an ethical analysis. *Journal of Neuroscience*, 28(19), 4841–3, https://doi.org/10.1523/JNEUROSCI.1493-08.2008

14. Edelson et al. (2011), Following the crowd, 110

15. Ibid., 111

16. Mildner, J. N. & Tamir, D. I. (2021). The people around you are inside your head: Social context shapes spontaneous thought. *Journal of Experimental Psychology: General*, 150(11), 2375–86, https://doi.org/10.1037/xge0001057

17. Mar, R. A. et al. (2012). How daydreaming relates to life satisfaction, loneliness, and social support: The importance of gender and daydream content. *Consciousness and Cognition*, 21(1), 401–7.

18. Song, X. & Wang, X. (2012). Mind wandering in Chinese daily lives – an experience sampling study. *PLOS ONE*, 7, e44423.

19. Gazzaniga, M. (2008). The Seed Salon: Tom Wolfe + Michael Gazzaniga, transcribed at https://2thinkgood.com/2008/07/01/tom-wolfe-seed-interview/

20. https://www.bls.gov/opub/ted/2021/time-spent-alone-increased-by-an-hour-per-day-in-2020.htm; note, the data also show that the pandemic has resulted in people spending more time alone, at least during 2020.

21. Dunbar, R. I. et al. (1997). Human conversational behavior. *Human Nature*, 8(3), 231–46.

22. https://www.tandfonline.com/doi/pdf/10.1080/03637759009376202; Vangelisti, Anita L. et al. (1990). Conversational narcissism. *Communication Monographs*, 57(4), 251–74, https://doi.org/10.1080/03637759009376202 – small-scale study indicating that narcissists try to focus conversation on themselves.

23. Tamir, D. I. and Mitchell, J. P. (2012). Disclosing information about the self is intrinsically rewarding. *Proceedings of the National Academy of Sciences*, 109, 8038–43.

24. Baek, E. C. et al. (2021). Activity in the brain's valuation and mentalizing networks is associated with propagation of online recommendations. *Scientific Reports*, 11(1), 1–11, https://www.nature.com/articles/s41598-021-90420-2

25. Rossignac-Milon, M. et al. (2021). Merged minds: Generalized shared reality in dyadic relationships. *Journal of Personality and Social Psychology*, 120(4), 882, https://cuhigginslab.com/publications/

26. Ibid.

27. Obama, Barack (2020). *A Promised Land*. Penguin, p. 52.

28. Galeotti, Mark (2022). *A Short History of Russia*. Penguin.

29. Yamashiro, J. K. & Hirst, W. (2020). Convergence on collective memories: Central speakers and distributed remembering. *Journal of Experimental Psychology: General*, 149(3), 461.

7: WE USE CONVERSATIONS TO CREATE OUR CULTURES

1. Wrangham, R.W., Wilson, M.L. & Muller, M.N. (2006). Comparative rates of violence in chimpanzees and humans. *Primates*, 47, 14–26, https://doi.org/10.1007/s10329-005-0140-1

2. https://quoteinvestigator.com/tag/charles-de-gaulle/

3. Wiesel, Elie (2008). A God Who Remembers, on *All Things Considered*, https://www.npr.org/2008/04/07/89357808/a-god-who-remembers?t=1632475811284

4. Vargha-Khadem, Faraneh, Gadian, David G. and Mishkin, Mortimer (2001). Dissociations in cognitive memory: the syndrome of developmental amnesia. *Philosophical Transactions of the Royal Society B: Biological Sciences*, 356(1413), 1435–40, https://royalsocietypublishing.org/doi/abs/10.1098/rstb.2001.0951

5. Graeber, D. & Wengrow, D. (2021). *The Dawn of Everything: A New History of Humanity*. Penguin. Although controversial, this monograph should at least upset any linear theory of progression from a pre-agricultural arcadia, through agriculture and onwards inevitably to modernism. While an exhilarating read, it fails to answer its own question regarding why other futures haven't come to be, and why we're almost locked into particular ways of organising our social orders.

6. Kashima, Y. (2008). A social psychology of cultural dynamics: Examining how cultures are formed, maintained, and transformed. *Social and Personality Psychology Compass*, 2(1), 107–20.

7. Ibid., 108.

8. Festinger, L. et al. (2017/1956). *When Prophecy Fails: A Social and Psychological Study of a Modern Group that Predicted the Destruction of the World*. Morrisville, NC: Lulu Press. Introduction at http://palimpsest.stmarytx.edu/thanneken/th7391/primary/FestingerEtAl(1956)WhenProphecyFails.pdf

9. https://www.nytimes.com/2007/10/08/opinion/08mon4.html

10. Of course, the great empires of the past propagated their own culture into a new setting, often with enduring consequences.

11. Yamashiro, J. K. & Roediger, H. L. (2021). Biased collective memories and historical overclaiming: An availability heuristic account. *Memory & Cognition*, 49(2), 311–22.

12. Ibid.

13. https://en.wikipedia.org/wiki/Culture_war

14. https://www.theguardian.com/world/2021/jun/13/everything-you-wanted-to-know-about-the-culture-wars-but-were-afraid-to-ask

15. https://www.theguardian.com/commentisfree/2021/may/24/oriel-college-rhodes-statue-anti-racist-anger

16. There is a debate over whether Cromwell ever uttered this exact phrase, and I am not a professional historian, and so can't, and won't, adjudicate. Wikipedia notes: 'In Irish popular memory of the Cromwellian Plantation, the Commonwealth is said to have declared that all the Catholic Irish must "go to Hell or to Connaught", west of the River Shannon. However, according to historian Padraig Lenihan, "The Cromwellians did not proclaim 'To Hell or to Connaught'. Connaught was chosen as a native reservation not because the land was poor; the Commonwealth rated Connaught above Ulster in this respect." Lenihan suggests that County Clare was chosen instead for security reasons – to keep Catholic landowners penned between the sea and the River Shannon.' Nevertheless, 'The Cromwellian transplantation is often cited as an early modern example of ethnic cleansing,' https://en.wikipedia.org/wiki/Act_for_the_Settlement_of_Ireland_1652. Winston Churchill (in his *A History of the English-Speaking Peoples*) was to describe Cromwell's record in Ireland as a 'lasting bane', concluding that 'Upon all of us there still lies "the curse of Cromwell".'

17. The article (https://www.theatlantic.com/newsletters/archive/2021/06/atlantic-daily-how-to-understand-boris-johnson/619126/, dated June 2021) is headed 'Boris Johnson Knows Exactly What He's Doing'; however, confusing a person's psychological certainty and self-belief with their epistemic contact with external reality is a common error. As of this writing (January 2023), the headline's claim has proven incorrect, and Johnson is currently two prime ministers ago. See this piece from the same source (January 2022): https://www.theatlantic.com/ideas/archive/2022/01/boris-johnson-winston-churchill/621294/, and (ahem) https://www.theatlantic.com/international/archive/2022/01/boris-johnson-party-pressure/621325/

18. Mokyr, Joel (2015). 2015 Balzan Prize for Economic History, https://www.balzan.org/en/prizewinners/joel-mokyr/acceptance-speech/; O'Brien, Dan (2022). Census confirms that reports of the death of rural Ireland are greatly exaggerated, https://www.businesspost.ie/analysis-opinion/dan-obrien-census-confirms-that-reports-of-the-death-of-rural-ireland-are-greatly-exaggerated/ (Ireland has not had much of a happy past, and O'Brien, noting Mokyr's comment, says there is 'less nostalgia for an illusory halcyon past in Ireland' with few attempts to weaponise nostalgia).

19. Turner, J. R. & Stanley, J. T. (2021). Holding on to pieces of the past: Daily reports of nostalgia in a life-span sample. *Emotion*, 21, 951–61, https://doi.org/10.1037/emo0000980

20. https://www.persuasion.community/p/-the-weaponization-of-nostalgia

21. Merck, C. et al. (2016). Collective mental time travel: Creating a shared future through our shared past. *Memory Studies*, 9(3), 284–94.

22. Hirst and Coman (2018), Building a collective memory.

23. Sequeira, S., Nunn, N. and Qian, N. (2020). Immigrants and the Making of America. *Review of Economic Studies*, 87, 382–419, https://doi.org/10.1093/restud/rdz003. They report that 'Counties with more historical immigration have higher incomes, less unemployment, less poverty, more education, and higher shares of urban population. We also found that these economic benefits do not have long-run social costs.'

24. Portes, J. (2019). The Economics of Migration. *Contexts*, 18, 12–17, https://journals.sagepub.com/doi/full/10.1177/1536504219854712

8: OUR NATIONS BEGAN AS CONVERSATIONS: COUNTRIES ARE COGNITIVE CONSTRUCTS

1. Atran (2022), The will to fight.

2. Examples include the Common Travel Area between the UK and Ireland, or the Schengen Area within the European Union.

3. Fiske, S. T. (2010). Envy up, scorn down: how comparison divides us. *American Psychologist*, 65, 698, https://www.ncbi.nlm.nih.gov/pmc/articles/PMC3825032/

4. https://www.npr.org/sections/goatsandsoda/2019/06/14/730257541/countries-are-ranked-on-everything-from-health-to-happiness-whats-the-point; https://www.ted.com/talks/simon_anholt_which_country_does_the_most_good_for_the_world/transcript

5. The whole 'my passport is better because we changed the colour of the cover' debate in the UK in 2019 was a most curious affair to an outside onlooker, especially as the colour of the cover was never mandated to begin with.

6. https://biblehub.com/deuteronomy/27-17.htm

7. Abel, M., Umanath, S., Fairfield, B., Takahashi, M., Roediger III, H. L. & Wertsch, J. V. (2019). Collective memories across 11 nations for World War II: Similarities and differences regarding the most important events. *Journal of Applied Research in Memory and Cognition*, 8(2), 178–88.

8. Roediger and Abel (2015), Collective memory.

9. Yes, this is pointed at certain Brexity types, and their laboured imaginations bringing forth a mouse.

10. https://en.wikipedia.org/wiki/B%C3%BCsingen_am_Hochrhein

11. https://en.wikipedia.org/wiki/India%E2%80%93Bangladesh_enclaves: Wiki summarises the situation as follows 'The main body of Bangladesh contained 102 Indian enclaves, which in turn contained 21 Bangladeshi counter-enclaves, one of which contained Dahala Khagrabari, an Indian counter-counter-enclave, the world's only third-order enclave when it existed. The Indian mainland contained 71 Bangladeshi enclaves, which in turn contained 3 Indian counter-enclaves.'

12. https://www.brookings.edu/blog/up-front/2020/05/12/sambandh-blog-india-and-bangladesh-exchanging-border-enclaves-re-connecting-with-new-citizens/

13. Wiki lists many: https://en.wikipedia.org/wiki/List_of_territorial_disputes

14. Roediger and Abel (2015), Collective memory.

15. DeScioli, P. (2023). On the origin of laws by natural selection. *Evolution and Human Behavior*, https://doi.org/10.1016/j.evolhumbehav.2023.01.004

16. Prado, M. & Trebilcock, M. (2009). Path dependence, development, and the dynamics of institutional reform. *University of Toronto Law Journal*, 59(3), 341–80.

17. I emphasise the complexity of Burke's origin for a reason: personal identities (indeed family histories) are not simple, even if the unthinking wish them so. Knowing the complexity of origins blunts attempts at appropriation of individuals to a cause or a country. There is a fine statue of Burke at the entrance to Trinity College Dublin, where I work; Burke was a Trinity undergraduate (see also this excellent Twitter thread on Burke's origins by Dr Anne Marie D'Arcy: https://twitter.com/dramdarcy/status/1448803821833146371).

18. Anderson led a more complicated life than Burke: his full name was Benedict Richard O'Gorman Anderson (1936–2015), born in China to an Anglo-Irish father and an English mother, brought up in Waterford, later educated in England (Eton and Cambridge), and subsequently lived in the USA (Cornell), where he became a renowned scholar of south-east Asia. His autobiography (*A Life Beyond Boundaries: A Memoir*, 2016) is a delight.

19. Anderson, B. (2006). *Imagined Communities: Reflections on the Origin and Spread of Nationalism*. Verso Books. As of this writing (January 2023), Google Scholar records about 137,000 citations to this book – a staggering number indeed, as most academics would be delighted with thirty-seven citations to a single item of their work (https://scholar.google.com/scholar?cites=13512913374545888922&as_sdt=2005&sciodt=0,5&hl=en).

20. Anderson (2006), *Imagined Communities*, p. 6.

21. De Gaulle's first broadcast to France, 18 June 1940, https://www.bbc.com/historyofthebbc/anniversaries/june/de-gaulles-first-broadcast-to-france/#:~:text=At%2010pm%20on%2018%20June,Resistance%20to%20him%20in%20London

22. Anderson (2006), *Imagined Communities*, p. 6.

23. Ibid., p. 140.

24. Margulis, E. H., Wong, P. C., Turnbull, C., Kubit, B. M. & McAuley, J. D. (2022). Narratives imagined in response to instrumental music reveal culture-bounded inter-subjectivity. *Proceedings of the National Academy of Sciences*, 119(4), e2110406119.

25. Anderson (2006), *Imagined Communities*, p. 37.

26. Mulhall, Daniel (2015). 'W. B. Yeats and the Ireland of his time', a talk delivered at the Oxford Literary Festival, https://www.dfa.ie/irish-embassy/great-britain/news-and-events/2015/wb-yeats-and-the-ireland-of-his-time/

27. There's a huge literature on this topic, and I'm certainly no expert on it; I have relied on Pine, L. (2010). *Education in Nazi Germany*. Bloomsbury. The following academic paper reminds me of the movie *Raiders of the Lost Ark*: Arnold, B. (2006). 'Arierdämmerung': race and archaeology in Nazi Germany. *World Archaeology*, 38(1), 8–31. And see Saini, A. (2019). *Superior: The Return of Race Science*. 4th Estate. I sometimes wonder how Nazis would reconcile modern genomics and archaeology unequivocally demonstrating our very human out-of-Africa origin with their beliefs; I assume they would resort to condemning 'degenerate' science or some such.

28. It is remarkable the extent to which it is not understood even by the members (and especially by a former member) that the EU is shared cognitive reality – a construct – imagined into existence by mutual agreement among the nation states, in their own national interests. Brussels has no armies, and can do nothing unless the member states agree to what it wants to do. Brussels has no authority other than the authority given to it willingly by the member states, and that ceded authority can be withdrawn if the member states so desire.

29. https://worldpopulationreview.com/country-rankings/newest-countries

9: IMAGINING OUR FUTURE NATIONS, TOGETHER

1. Dennett, D. C. (1995). Darwin's dangerous idea. *The Sciences*, 35(3), 34–40.

2. https://www.worldatlas.com/articles/how-many-languages-are-spoken-in-nyc.html; https://www.timeout.com/newyork/news/this-interactive-map-highlights-the-700-languages-spoken-in-nyc-041921

3. https://migrationobservatory.ox.ac.uk/resources/briefings/london-census-profile/

4. http://media.isnet.org/kmi/iptek/Darwin/Descent/chapter_05.html

5. https://www.mercatus.org/publications/government-spending/2-percent-growth-rate-it-would-take-35-years-double-size-us-economy

6. O'Brien, Ed (2022). Losing Sight of Piecemeal Progress: People Lump and Dismiss Improvement Efforts that Fall Short of Categorical Change – Despite Improving. *Psychological Science*, 33(8), 1278–99, https://journals.sagepub.com/doi/full/10.1177/09567976221075302

7. Mitchell, G. & Tetlock, P.E. (2022). Are Progressives in Denial about Progress? Yes, But So Is Almost Everyone Else. *Clinical Psychological Science*, 21677026221114315, https://journals.sagepub.com/doi/full/10.1177/21677026221114315

8. https://ourworldindata.org/

9. https://www.thecut.com/2017/01/why-being-part-of-a-crowd-feels-so-good.html

10. Gabriel et al. (2017). The psychological importance of collective assembly: Development and validation of the Tendency for Effervescent Assembly Measure (TEAM). *Psychological Assessment*, 29(11), 1349–62, https://doi.org/10.1037/pas 0000434, https://www.researchgate.net/publication/314271695_The_Psychological_ Importance_of_Collective_Assembly_Development_and_Validation_of_the_Tendency_ for_Effervescent_Assembly_Measure_TEAM

11. Martel, F. A. et al. (2021). Why True Believers Make the Ultimate Sacrifice: Sacred Values, Moral Convictions, or Identity Fusion? *Frontiers in Psychology*, 12:779120, https://doi.org/10.3389/fpsyg.2021.779120, PMID: 34867692, PMCID: PMC8634031.

12. Öztop, Fatma Anıl (2022). Motivational factors of Turkish foreign terrorist fighters in ISIS. *Middle Eastern Studies*, 58(4), 553–72, https://doi.org/10.1080/00263206.20 21.1978984

13. https://www.france24.com/en/europe/20220603-foreign-fighters-explain-motivations-for-joining-ukraine-s-war-effort; https://www.npr.org/2022/06/15/ 1105318161/whats-motivating-the-foreigners-who-have-gone-to-ukraine-to-fight-against-russia?t=1657196718219; I haven't been able to find a systematic empirical study addressing this issue, so these are really supportive anecdotes. And there may be other issues with foreign fighters (e.g. https://www.brookings.edu/blog/order-from-chaos/2022/03/03/foreign-fighters-in-ukraine-evaluating-the-benefits-and-risks/).

14. Higgins, Rossignac-Milon & Echterhoff (2021), Shared reality.

15. A saying attributed to Sir John Templeton, as the four most expensive words in the English language.

16. I have my peer-review publication scars, but they've been worth it: https://scholar. google.com/citations?user=tVnIUCUAAAAJ&hl=en

17. Topcu, M. N. & Hirst, W. (2020). Remembering a nation's past to imagine its future: The role of event specificity, phenomenology, valence, and perceived agency. *Journal of Experimental Psychology: Learning, Memory, and Cognition*, 46(3), 563.

18. Or at least Freud is regularly cited as having said this, e.g. https://www.themost10. com/engrossing-sigmund-freud-quotes/

19. Topcu & Hirst (2020), Remembering a nation's past to imagine its future. This study consisted of two experiments involving approximately 200 participants, ranging in age from twenty to seventy-three, with an average age of thirty-six to thirty-eight.

20. For each item generated, they requested a 1–7 rating of the sharpness, visual detail, sound detail, vividness, detailedness, location clarity, time clarity and comprehensibleness. Participants were also asked to indicate when the event(s) had occurred, how strongly they felt about the event(s), the extent to which they, others or circumstances had caused the events.

21. Topcu & Hirst (2020), Remembering a nation's past to imagine its future. Groupings were determined by agreement, when there was a high degree of inter-rater reliability.

22. Ibid., p. 575.

23. Ibid.

24. From Ernest Hemingway's *The Sun Also Rises* (1926).

25. Adolphs, R. (2009). The social brain: neural basis of social knowledge. *Annu. Rev. Psychol.*, 60, 693–716; Wagner, D. D. et al. (2012). The representation of self and person knowledge in the medial prefrontal cortex. *Wiley Interdisciplinary Reviews: Cognitive Science*, 3, 451–70; Yeshurun, Y., Nguyen, M. & Hasson, U. (2021). The default mode network: where the idiosyncratic self meets the shared social world. *Nature Reviews Neuroscience*, 22(3), 181–92.

26. Gagnepain, P. et al. (2020). Collective memory shapes the organization of individual memories in the medial prefrontal cortex. *Nature Human Behaviour*, 4(2), 189–200.

27. Halbwachs, M. (1992). *On Collective Memory*. University of Chicago Press, p. 42

28. Gagnepain et al. (2020), Collective memory shapes the organization of individual memories in the medial prefrontal cortex, p. 9

29. Aggleton & O'Mara (2022), The anterior thalamic nuclei.

30. Wertsch, J. V. & Roediger III, H. L. (2008). Collective memory: Conceptual foundations and theoretical approaches. *Memory*, 16(3), 318–26, https://www.tandfonline.com/doi/full/10.1080/09658210701801434

31. Macron admits French forces 'tortured and murdered' Algerian freedom fighter, https://www.france24.com/en/france/20210303-france-algeria-macron-admits-torture-freedom-fighter

32. Barbero, M. (2021). France Still Struggles with the Shadow of the 'War without a Name', https://foreignpolicy.com/2021/02/13/france-algerian-war-legacy-politics-colonialism/

33. Stone, C. B. et al. (2017). Forgetting history: The mnemonic consequences of listening to selective recountings of history. *Memory Studies*, 10, 286–96, https://journals.sagepub.com/doi/full/10.1177/1750698017701610

34. Ibid., 288.

35. Ibid., 291.

36. https://literature.stackexchange.com/questions/20248/who-said-that-history-is-a-lie-fable-agreed-upon

37. Edmund Burke: Reflections on the Revolution in France (1790), https://cyber.harvard.edu/bridge/Philosophy/burke.htm

AFTERWORD

1. https://www.irishtimes.com/news/politics/furious-response-to-column-saying-ireland-has-tenuous-claim-to-nationhood-1.3001173

2. https://www.thejc.com/lets-talk/all/ukraine-shows-how-vital-the-nation-is-in-defending-freedom-5Y8BzbUg3UE5VFWRIS79kx. Don't expect any intellectual consistency between these stances.

3. This piece is truly astounding: https://www.rte.ie/brainstorm/2022/0511/1297303-ireland-britain-sinn-fein-conservatives-imperialism/; it is by a professor of politics at Queen's University, Belfast. But he is not alone. Another professor of history (at Cambridge University), pumped up on the sugar-rush of Brexitism, tells us that 'The EU may be a club ... but it should never forget that the Anglo-Americans own the freehold of the property on which the club is built. Brussels and the continental capitals are at best leaseholders' (https://www.newstatesman.com/world/2017/03/world-after-brexit); note, this latter historian also thinks that King Charles III should be made 'Emperor of Europe' (https://engelsbergideas.com/notebook/charles-iii-why-not-make-him-king-emperor-of-europe/).

4. Melzer, Richard (1998). Review in *Journal of American History*, 85, 1179–80.

5. Accampo, Elinor (2015). Review in *Journal of Modern History*, 87(4), 938–41.

6. Quoted in Wilson, Conor (2022). 'Pandemics don't end with a bang' – lessons from the Spanish Flu, https://www.rte.ie/news/primetime/2022/0125/1275848-spanish-flu-lessons-covid-19/

INDEX